ANATOMICAL BASIS OF CARDIAC INTERVENTIONS, VOLUME 2

Kalyanam Shivkumar, MD, PhD, Series Editor

Atlas of
INTERVENTIONAL
ELECTROPHYSIOLOGY

Roderick Tung, MD

Shumpei Mori, MD, PhD

Kalyanam Shivkumar, MD, PhD

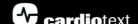

Cardiotext Publishing, LLC
750 2nd St NE Suite 102
Hopkins, Minnesota 55343
USA

www.cardiotextpublishing.com

Any updates to this book may be found at: https://cardiotextpublishing.com/electrophysiology-heart
-rhythm-mgmt/atlas-of-interventional-electrophysiology

Comments, inquiries, and requests for bulk sales can be directed to the publisher at: info@cardiotext
publishing.com.

Library of Congress Control Number: 2024933619

ISBN: 978-1-942909-60-6

eISBN: 978-1-942909-66-8

Printed in the United States of America

2 3 4 5 6 7 8   29 28 27 26 25 24

With deepest gratitude to Meyer and Renée Luskin for their
kind and generous support in publishing this volume.

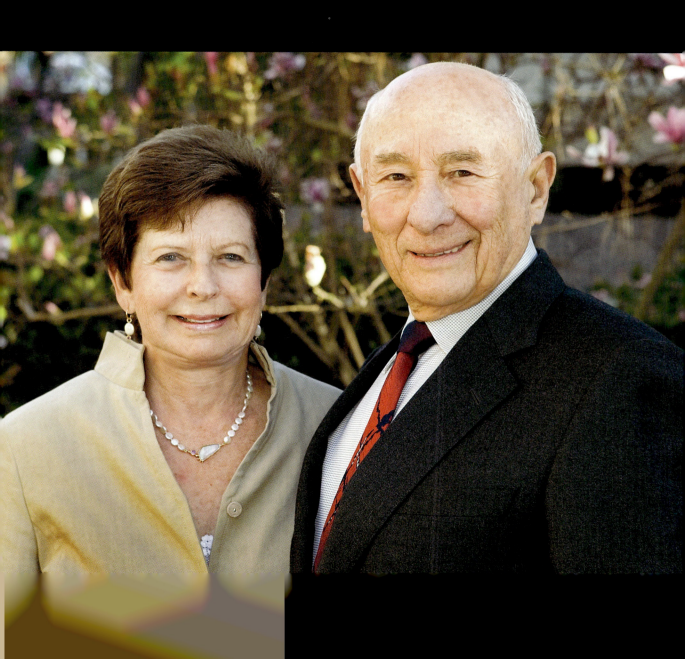

The *Atlas of Interventional Electrophysiology* is *Volume 2* in the *Anatomical Basis of Cardiac Intervention* series, which represents a significant milestone for the Amara Yad Project.

The origin of the Amara Yad Project, which is best viewed as a knowledge portal, can be traced back to 2012 when our journey toward establishing a new gold standard in anatomical textbooks commenced.

At that time, we uncovered the disturbing history of the Pernkopf atlases, which had been held in high regard. The impetus was to surpass that work and thereby honor the memories of the victims of the Nazi regime who were subjects of those infamous atlases. Our project included identifying several material resources, funding, and assembling a team of experts to develop a new generation of atlases.

In parallel, we fine-tuned several experimental methods to prepare specimens that allowed us to chart the entire human body. The heart was the first part of human anatomy chosen for study, mainly inspired by our clinical specialization and research focus. The catalyst for the effort was the great fortune of locating the Wallace A. McAlpine Collection, its subsequent acquisition, and digitization for its use in this effort.

Over the years, many trainees and colleagues we have interacted with at UCLA and elsewhere in the world have encouraged and fiercely supported this effort by our group. Indeed, it has been gratifying to note that several scientific publications now use content from these new atlases to disseminate anatomical information relating to the heart. The journey to map the entire human body is well underway and will involve internationally recognized experts who will author individual volumes of the series.

Two renowned experts, Drs. Roderick Tung and Shumpei Mori, have joined me in preparing *Volume 2* of the series relating to the heart. Over the years at the UCLA Cardiac Arrhythmia Center, Drs. Tung and Mori particularly stand out for their passion for anatomy and enthusiasm for this project. Their dedication to science, passion for teaching, artistic flair, and attention to detail will be evident to any reader perusing *Volume 2*. It has been a special privilege to work with them on this volume.

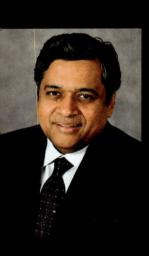

Kalyanam Shivkumar, MD, PhD

Professor of Medicine (Cardiology), Radiology & Bioengineering
Director, UCLA Cardiac Arrhythmia Center & EP Programs
Director & Chief, Cardiovascular & Interventional Programs
David Geffen School of Medicine & UCLA Health System
Los Angeles, California

Dr. Shivkumar is a physician scientist serving as the inaugural director of the UCLA Cardiac Arrhythmia Center & EP Programs (since its establishment in 2002) and as the Director and Chief of UCLA's Cardiovascular & Interventional Programs. He leads a team that provides state-of-the-art clinical care and has developed several innovative therapies for the non-pharmacological management of cardiac arrhythmias and other cardiac diseases. He has a long track record of research publications and books. He has been elected as a member of the American Society of Clinical Investigation (ASCI), the Association of American Physicians (AAP), the Association of University Cardiologists (AUC) and is an honorary fellow of the Royal College of Physicians, London (FRCP). He currently serves as the Editor-in-Chief of the *Journal of the American College of Cardiology: Clinical Electrophysiology*.

Dedication

To the Past, Present, and Future of the Tung family: Mom and Dad, Patricia and Theodore, for teaching me love and the rewards of a relentless work ethic. My sister, Candice, who is my best friend and life mentor. My wife, Ewelina, for believing in our shared vision and showing me new depths of love that continue to grow. My son, Alex, and daughter, Eliana, you fill our hearts with immense joy, pride, and optimism.

To gratitude for life, love, art, and science—for that is the human experience.

—Roderick Tung

To my wife, Hwaryung, and our children, Toshitada and Toshiteru.
To my parents, Toshihiko and Ruriko Mori, and my sisters, Satoko and Naoko.

—Shumpei Mori

To the memory of my beloved parents, Ramanathan Kalyanam Iyer (1932–1992) and Saraswathi Venkataraman Iyer (1934–2020). To my wife, Preethi, our son, Tejas, and my sister, Nitya Kalyani.

—Kalyanam Shivkumar

ONLINE ACCESS

The purchase of a new copy of this book entitles the first retail purchaser to free personal online access to a digital version of this edition.

Please send a copy of your purchase receipt to info@cardiotext.com with subject ATLAS V2 EBOOK, and we will email you a redemption code along with instructions on how to access the digital file.

Table of Contents

Acknowledgments

We would like to thank the family of Dr. Wallace A. McAlpine—his daughters Ms. Laurel Flowers, Ms. Kim Renteria Clark, and Ms. Leigh McAlpine Whitten, and his son, Mr. Fraser McAlpine—for helping us locate Dr. McAlpine's works. In 2013, Dr. Bruce Lytle at the Cleveland Clinic helped locate the physical collection, and subsequently, the collection was officially transferred to UCLA for the multi-year digitization project. We gratefully acknowledge the Cleveland Clinic Foundation for this gesture. We would also like to acknowledge the Leonetti O'Connell Foundation and Dr. Craig Gordon for their unrestricted gifts for the development of *Volume 1* in the series *Anatomical Basis of Cardiac Interventions*, which paved the way to make this expensive project a reality.

This project also made it obvious to us that it is a true privilege to be part of a team at UCLA with inspiring colleagues. Our electrophysiology mentor, Professor Noel G. Boyle, deserves special mention for encouraging us to pursue this project in the first place. We thank all the faculty, staff, and trainees at the UCLA Cardiac Arrhythmia Center, UCLA Cardiac Interventional Programs, and the UCLA Departments of Surgery and Radiology for our useful interactions. The interactions and feedback from our exceptional trainees over the years at UCLA are much appreciated. Special thanks to Dr. Takanori Sato for his support during photo sessions. We thank our colleague Professor Olujimi A. Ajijola, who paved the way for this work with his expert oversight of the scientific core lab and for establishing and maintaining a human heart pipeline for research.

We would like to express our deep gratitude to the selfless individuals who have donated their bodies and tissues for the advancement of education and research. This project was supported by the UCLA Amara Yad Project. Special thanks to One Legacy Foundation and the NIH SPARC Program, which formed the basis for obtaining donor hearts for research and for funding this effort. We appreciate our Research Operations Manager, Amiksha S. Gandhi for her dedication to support our projects. Special thanks to the Surgical Sciences Laboratory at UCLA (Professor Warwick J. Peacock and Dr. Grace Chang). We are grateful to Professor Michael C. Fishbein at the Department of Pathology and Laboratory Medicine at UCLA for his valuable guidance, and to all the staff members of the UCLA Donated Body Program, Translational Research Imaging Center (Department of Radiology) at UCLA, and Translational Pathology Core Laboratory at UCLA. We thank Ms. Michelle Betwarda at the UCLA Cardiac Arrhythmia Center for her administrative acumen and tenacity, which ensured the acquisition and digitization of the McAlpine Collection.

We thank Mr. Michael Papalucas, who expertly digitized the original slides made by Dr. McAlpine. We are grateful to Dr. Hatsue Ishibashi-Ueda at Hokusetsu General Hospital, Professor Taka-aki Matsuyama at Showa University School of Medicine, and Ms. Diane E. Spicer at the Heart Institute at Johns Hopkins All Children's Hospital and at the University of Florida for their guidance on pressure perfusion–fixation.

We thank Professor Venkat N. Tholakanahalli at the University of Minnesota, Professor Koji Fukuzawa and Dr. Kazutaka Nakasone at Kobe University Graduate School of Medicine, and Dr. Wei-Hsin Chung at China Medical University Hospital for supplying clinical images. Computed tomographic images were reconstructed using a commercially available workstation (Ziostation2, version 2.9.8.4; AMIN Co, Ltd; Ziosoft Inc.). The authors thank Yuki Inoue and Kingo Shichinohe at AMIN Co., Ltd., for their technical support. We appreciate the patience, dedication, and expertise provided by Cardiotext Publishing and the team led by Mr. Mike Crouchet for the output that is "bespoke" for this volume. Special thanks to Professors Kenneth A. Ellenbogen and Francis E. Marchlinski for their encouragement and for graciously writing the forewords for this book, and Dr. Andre d'Avila and Dr. Fermin C. Garcia for graciously providing their short comments for this book.

—Roderick Tung, MD
—Shumpei Mori, MD, PhD
—Kalyanam Shivkumar, MD, PhD

About the Authors

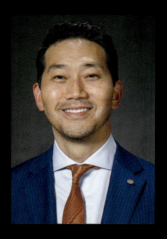

Roderick Tung, MD

Professor of Medicine
Chief, Division of Cardiology
Director, Banner Heart Institute
Director, Cardiovascular Clinical Research
The University of Arizona College of Medicine
Phoenix, Arizona

Dr. Tung is an internationally recognized clinical cardiologist, cardiac electrophysiologist, researcher, and educator. He received combined training in electrophysiology at Beth Israel Deaconess–Harvard Medical School with Mark Josephson and at UCLA David Geffen School of Medicine with Kalyanam Shivkumar. It was during his eight years at the UCLA Cardiac Arrhythmia Center that he was first exposed to the works of Wallace McAlpine and the planning of volumes of this Atlas collection. After serving as the director of the Center for Arrhythmia Care at the University of Chicago for over five years, he was recruited by the University of Arizona College of Medicine in Phoenix. His current vision as the Chief of Cardiology and Director of the Banner—University Medicine Heart Institute in Phoenix is to create a premier cardiovascular destination in the Southwest United States through programs of distinction and innovation. He has published over 270 peer-reviewed articles and continues to serve as the section editor for the *Journal of the American College of Cardiology: Clinical Electrophysiology* and *Heart Rhythm Journal*. He is the founding executive producer of *Heart Rhythm TV*, which aims to globalize education and advance the missions of the Heart Rhythm Society.

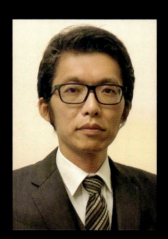

Shumpei Mori, MD, PhD

Adjunct Associate Professor of Medicine
Director, Specialized Program for Anatomy & Imaging
UCLA Cardiac Arrhythmia Center
David Geffen School of Medicine & UCLA Health System
Los Angeles, California

Dr. Mori is a physician scientist who serves as the Director of the Specialized Program for Anatomy & Imaging at UCLA Cardiac Arrhythmia Center. His field of specialization is cardiac anatomy and advanced clinical imaging. He has a long track record of publications and has published several books. In 2022, he co-authored *Volume 1* of this project, *Atlas of Cardiac Anatomy*. He is an editor of *Clinical Anatomy* and section editor at the *Journal of the American College of Cardiology: Clinical Electrophysiology*.

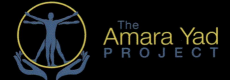

Amara Yad (The Immortal Hand) is a physician-led initiative with a single goal: To honor the victims of medical exploitation through corrective action. As its first act, Amara Yad will publish a new generation of open-access digital anatomic atlases of the highest quality. These digital atlases will be made available gratis to all users to support the life-saving mission of the profession, made possible with the generous backing of the Amara Yad Project initiated by the UCLA Cardiac Arrhythmia Center in 2022.

THE HISTORY

Between 1938 and the end of World War II, University of Vienna anatomist Eduard Pernkopf published a series of anatomical atlases. He used the bodies of over 1,300 murdered victims of Nazi terror as subjects for his work.

The Nazi history of the Pernkopf atlas series was concealed in the 1950s. Swastikas and SS insignia proudly displayed in the illustrators' signatures of those atlases were erased (partially) from prints in subsequent editions of the atlases. For decades, physicians used Pernkopf's atlases without the knowledge that bodies depicted in those works belonged to the victims of Nazi atrocities. The atlases were regarded as preeminent anatomical resources, a clinical necessity, and remained in use even after their depraved origins had been exposed. Importantly, no effort was made to surpass this work and provide a definitive resource for the world.

TODAY

Anatomic atlases are an indispensable resource for medical professionals. At UCLA, the production of clear and accurate atlases that support the lifesaving mission of the profession is made possible by the University's Willed Body Donor Program, U.S. federal research support for science, financial gifts from donors, and volunteer efforts of students and faculty.

We dedicate this second volume of the Amara Yad Project to the noble humans who have so generously willed their bodies for science and education. We also specifically honor the victims of medical exploitation in Pernkopf's atlases. We shift the focus away from the images of their bodies and toward their enduring human dignity.

Foreword

Cardiac anatomy is the core of what every cardiologist does and needs to know. In the *Atlas of Interventional Electrophysiology*, the second volume of the Amara Yad project, authors Roderick Tung, Shumpei Mori, and Kalyanam Shivkumar take our understanding and appreciation of cardiac anatomy to the next level.

It is critical to understand basic anatomy, but that is only the first step. We work in a fluoroscopic or a minimal or zero-fluoroscopic environment, integrate and understand anatomy with other imaging techniques, and then combine this with electrophysiologic recordings. For electrophysiologists, having the imaging and anatomy combined and illustrated with multiple modalities, plus the electrophysiologic recordings, can only be described and appreciated as the complete package. The *Atlas of Interventional Electrophysiology* builds on the tremendous legacy of McAlpine's original atlas and curated images. The excellence of *Volume 1* is now brought "front and center" in *Volume 2* of the *Anatomical Basis of Cardiac Interventions* series.

Atlas of Interventional Electrophysiology is a gift to every cardiologist and electrophysiologist interested in understanding structure and function of anatomy and (electro)physiology. The caliber of these illustrations and explanations is truly spectacular. I say with great certainty that *Volume 2* will become the first book trainees, educators, allied professionals, and physicians at all levels will reach for when preparing for cases in the electrophysiology laboratory. This book is a masterpiece and must be on every electrophysiologist's bookshelf. It will assuredly become a classic and a "go-to" resource for all of us.

Drs. Tung, Mori, and Shivkumar have provided us with a new volume in the *Anatomical Basis of Cardiac Interventions* series that earns its place next to *Volume 1* because it advances and integrates what we do on a daily basis. This book can best be described by paraphrasing William Shakespeare: "it will never grow old or stale." It is a gift to our field, and I encourage anyone with an interest in electrophysiology to pick it up and read it.

—Kenneth A. Ellenbogen, MD

We have been anxiously awaiting *Volume 2* of the *Anatomical Basis of Cardiac Interventions* series after spending hours marveling at the organization and quality of the normal heart images and learning from the authors' expertise shared in *Volume 1*. This series takes off our blindfold and shines a bright light on the best path forward. The *Atlas of Interventional Electrophysiology* should be required reading and review for all those who desire to optimize success and avoid risks and collateral injury during interventional cardiac procedures. Review all the images carefully, read the accompanying text, and then, repeat the process! The exponential gains for the effort made in understanding the details and the nuance related to cardiac anatomy make every moment spent a gift. Drs. Tung, Mori, and Shivkumar deserve our congratulations and gratitude.

—Francis E. Marchlinski, MD

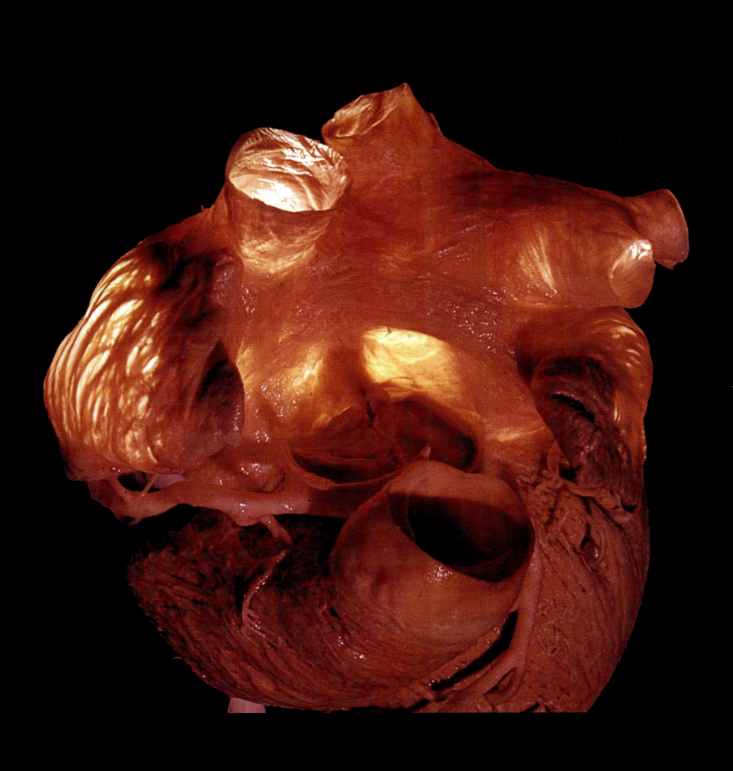

If there were one person, alive or dead, that we could meet, it would be Leonardo da Vinci. The consummate polymath, he embodied the thirst and passion to understand the human condition through both art and science. He was a philosopher, painter, sculptor, anatomist, theorist, inventor, and a student of the world. We currently live in a world that attempts to dichotomize this "right brain-left brain" duality that is unique to human nature. Yet, as humans, we cannot and should not accept categorization in such ways. The arts represent the desire to express our emotions and soul (to feel), and science represents our means to comprehend our universe (to understand) empirically and systematically.

In *Volume 2*, we build upon the fundamentals of *Volume 1* and apply both structural and functional concepts to the evolving practice of interventional cardiac electrophysiology. One cannot completely understand the precision needed to execute clinical procedures around complex anatomy without an appreciation of the human heart as an artistic form and structure. Our goal is to take you through a guided tour into and out of the heart, in the order of native blood flow while making the necessary stops to highlight clinical spotlights, where the understanding of regional anatomy is critical to both the safety and success of procedures performed throughout the world daily. We want the reader to have a 4D perspective while reading this *Atlas*, as if they are physically standing inside the heart section images displayed. What is below you? What is above you? What is to the left and right of you? The knowledge of regional anatomy enables the creative mind to understand vantage points to access challenging regions within the human heart.

The aesthetic of this volume is motivated by the desire to create a work that is equally deserving as an art book sitting on a coffee table or as a traditional upright on a bookshelf, as an anatomic reference. We purposely provide images without labels to allow the imagination to drift in wonderment, while at the same time forcing all students of anatomy to self-test by naming and identifying individual structures displayed. Every time we look at an image from the book, we should appreciate something new, as if we're seeing it for the first time, which should remind us of the infinite depths of understanding. This intersection between art and science is displayed with "mixed media" in *Volume 2*, with multimodality medical imaging of the same viewpoint with fluoroscopy, intracardiac echocardiography, 3D electroanatomic mapping, and schematics originally prepared by Dr. McAlpine.

We hope this *Atlas* fuels countless generations of learners and proceduralists, with patients and humankind as the global beneficiaries. This work has potential benefits across all levels of training and experience—from medical students, residents, and allied health professionals, to practicing interventional cardiologists, imaging specialists, and electrophysiologists. The investment into appreciating human anatomy is beyond a worthy endeavor, as the human form, as we know it, is highly unlikely to change over the next many thousands of years. We humbly submit this work to provide both clarity and inspiration to those who desire a fundamental yet deeper understanding of the beautiful field of cardiac electrophysiology through both art and science. We are always inspired by coach John Wooden to "make each day your masterpiece!"

—Roderick Tung, MD
—Shumpei Mori, MD, PhD
—Kalyanam Shivkumar, MD, PhD

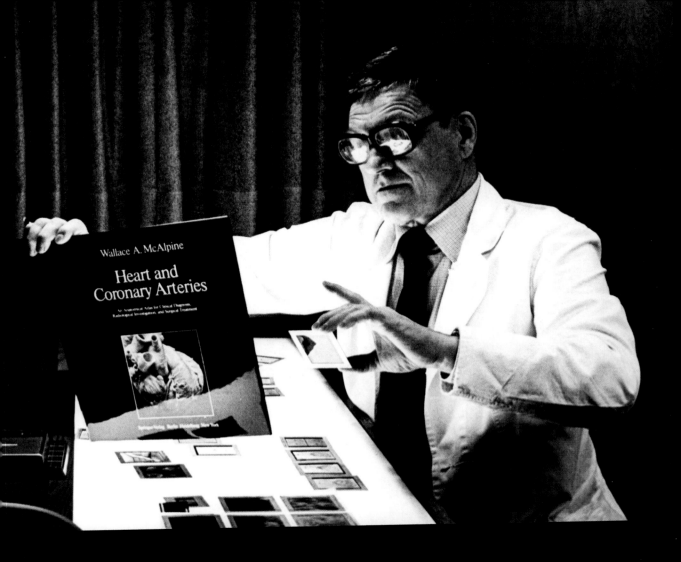

nowing anatomy well facilitates our learning and understanding of physiology . . . McAlpine
ictures and illustrations are incredibly didactic and will be the reference for both areas of medic
tudies for many years and greatly impact the present and future generations of electrophysio
gists and physicians in general.

—Andre d'Avila, MD, Ph

McAlpine's unique original work is a rich and thorough exploration of cardiac anatomy like neve
een before. It became an indispensable tool to understand interventional electrophysiologists
rocedures better. It is quite simple for me: there is before and after McAlpine.

Fermin C. Garcia M

In Memoriam

Wallace A. McAlpine, MD, FACS, FRCS (Eng), FRCS (Ed)
1920–2005

Dr. Wallace A. McAlpine's passion for cardiac anatomy and relentless attention to detail will continue to inspire and teach countless generations.

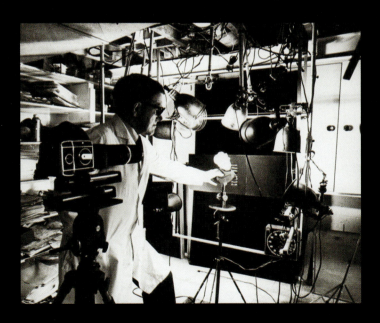
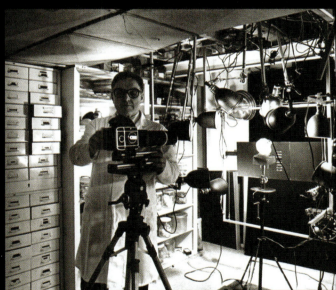

Terminology

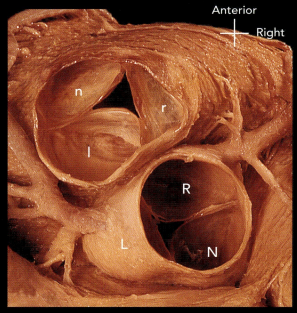

Anterior
Right

Terminology used in this textbook

Aortic root

R, right coronary aortic sinus/leaflet

L, left coronary aortic sinus/leaflet

N, noncoronary aortic sinus/leaflet

Pulmonary root

r, right adjacent (facing) pulmonary sinus/leaflet

l, left adjacent (facing) pulmonary sinus/leaflet

n, nonadjacent (facing) pulmonary sinus/leaflet

*The term cusp is currently used to indicate the sinus and/or leaflet in the clinical settings.

Attitudinal orientation
Aortic root
R, anterior
L, left posterior
N, right posterior

Pulmonary root
r, right anterior
l, posterior
n, left anterior

Nomina Anatomica
Aortic root
R, right
L, left
N, posterior/noncoronary

Pulmonary root
r, right
l, left
n, anterior

Terminologia Anatomica
Aortic root
R, right
L, left
N, noncoronary

Pulmonary root
r, right
l, left
n, anterior

Other abbreviations used in this text book)

RAO, right anterior oblique

LAO, left anterior oblique

LPO, left posterior oblique

List of Videos

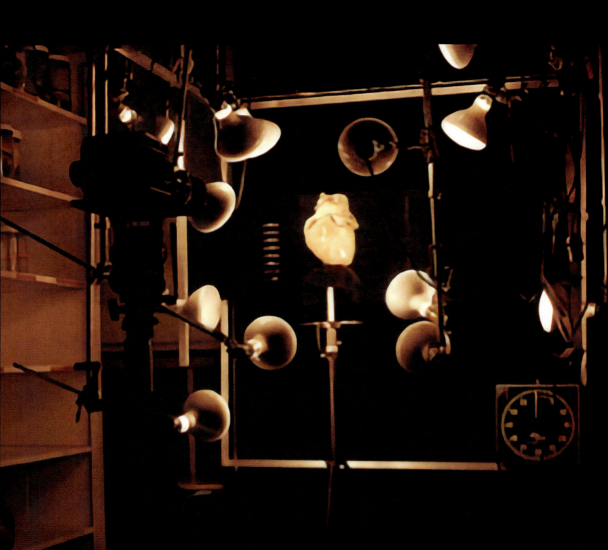

1

Cardiac Orientation

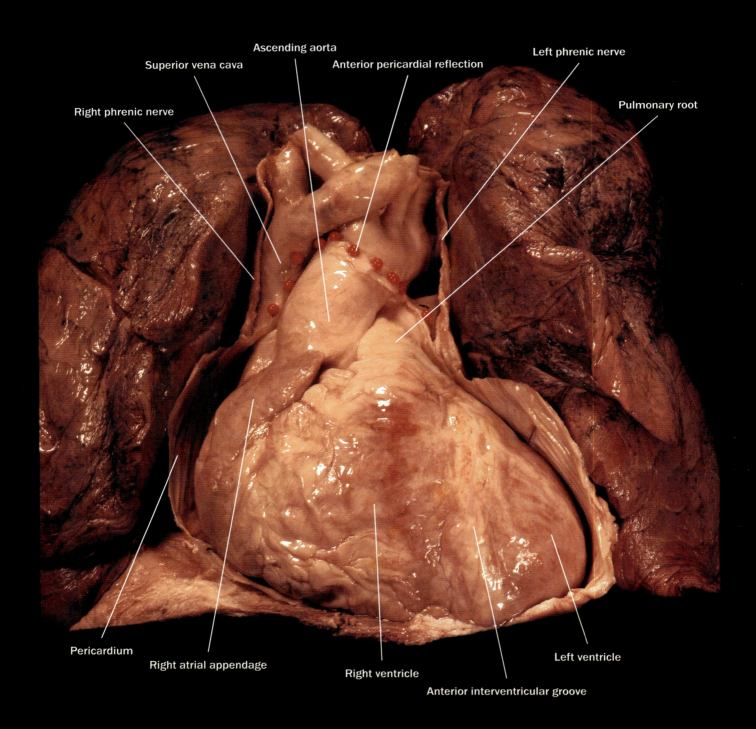

Right phrenic nerve

Superior vena cava

Ascending aorta

Anterior pericardial reflection

Left phrenic nerve

Pulmonary root

Pericardium

Right atrial appendage

Right ventricle

Anterior interventricular groove

Left ventricle

Figures 1-1 and 1-2   Frontal view of the heart in situ.

The importance of attitudinal views is highlighted by the in-situ anteroposterior view of the heart. The red pins indicate the most anterior and superior margins of the pericardial reflections.[1] Note that the aortic root and ascending aorta lie within the pericardial sac, which highlights the anatomic basis for pericardial tamponade from proximal aortic dissection. In this view, both left versus right and base versus apex are foreshortened. The anterior ventricle is the right ventricle.[2]

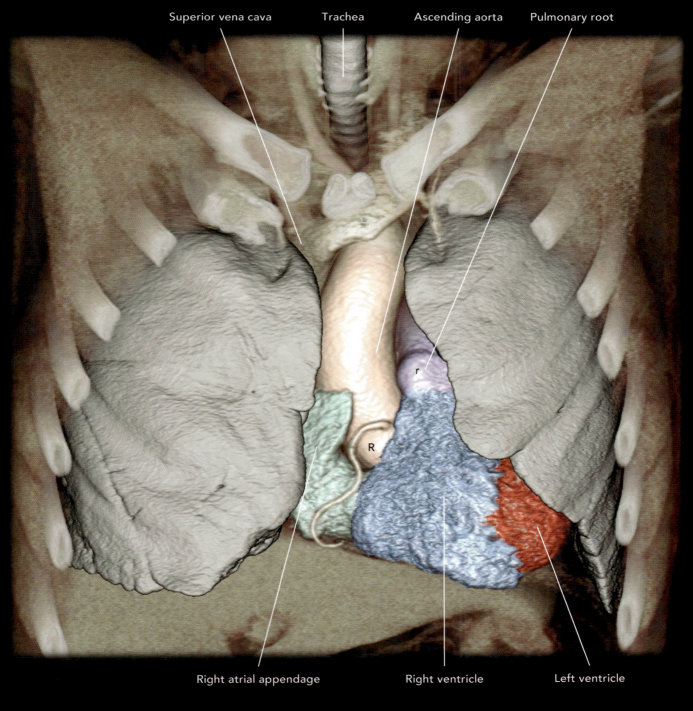

Superior vena cava   Trachea   Ascending aorta   Pulmonary root

Right atrial appendage   Right ventricle   Left ventricle

Part of the anterior and apical regions of the left ventricle can be observed from this direction. Thus, the left ventricle is leftward and posterior to the right ventricle. Mapping and ablation of the left ventricle requires reflecting the heart rightward and superiorly, or with insertion of catheters immediately leftward and posterior. The pulmonary artery is leftward of the aorta as it wraps around the aortic root. This explains the reversed points of auscultation (aortic murmurs from the right sternal border, and pulmonary murmurs from the left sternal border).

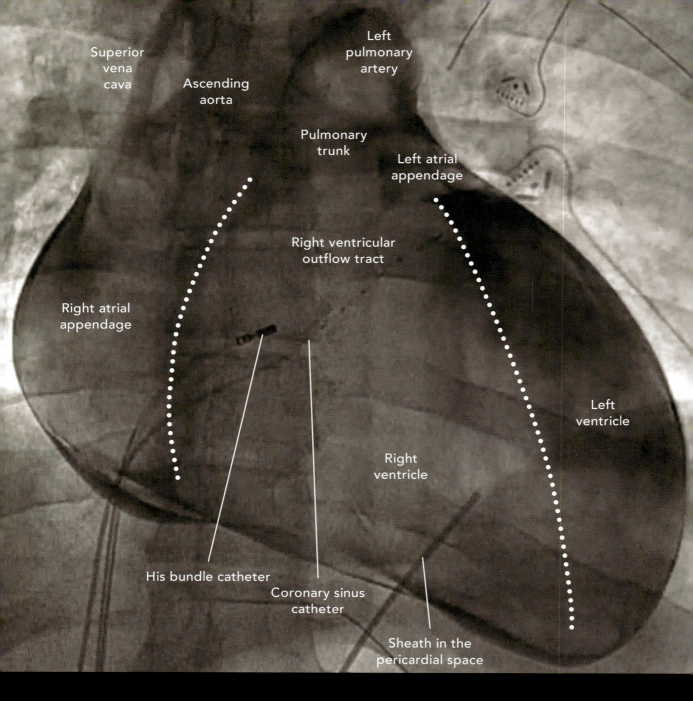

Figure 1-3 ▶ **and Figure 1-4** **Fluoroscopic correlation in the frontal view.**

The image is created by injection of contrast into the pericardial space. Standard His bundle and coronary sinus catheter positions are shown. The cardiac silhouette can be divided into thirds with the center depicting the right ventricle, the right atrium to the right, and the left ventricle to the left.

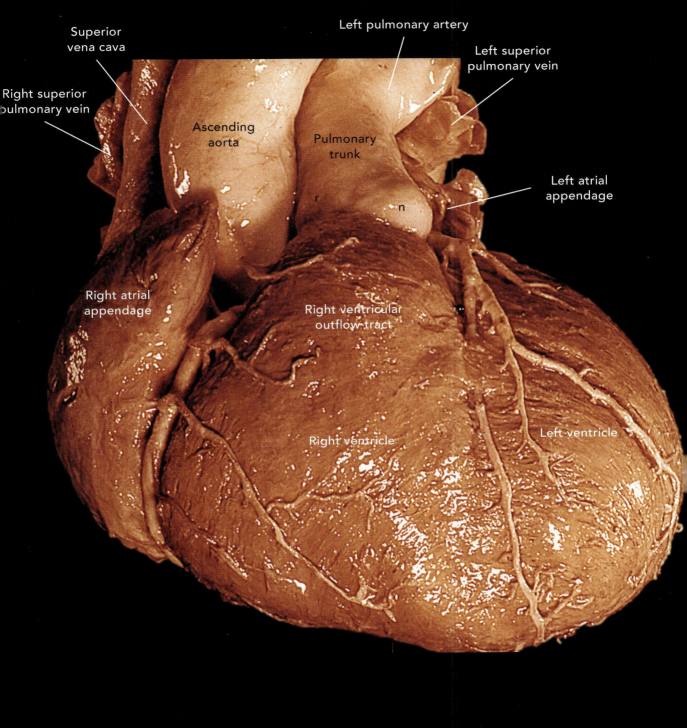

Superior
vena cava

Left pulmonary artery

Left superior
pulmonary vein

Right superior
pulmonary vein

Ascending
aorta

Pulmonary
trunk

r

n

Left atrial
appendage

Right atrial
appendage

Right ventricular
outflow tract

Right ventricle

Left ventricle

The left ventricle is represented by the left silhouette border, and the extent depends on the in-situ orientation and rotation of the heart. The tip of the left atrial appendage is seen at the superior left silhouette border adjacent to the pulmonary root/trunk. The right heart border consists entirely of the right atrium, specifically, the right atrial appendage.

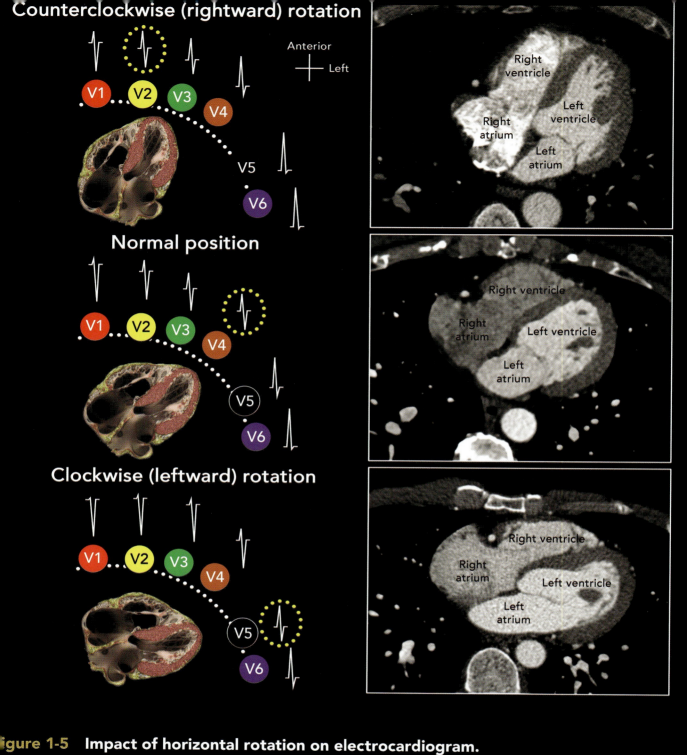

Figure 1-5 Impact of horizontal rotation on electrocardiogram.

The orientation of the heart within the thoracic cavity is variable. In patients with more clockwise (leftward) rotation, less of the left ventricle may be viewed from the frontal perspective. Conversely, in those with counterclockwise (rightward) rotation, a greater extent of the left ventricle will be represented as the left border of the cardiac silhouette in the frontal view. The 12-lead electrocardiogram will exhibit early precordial transition in counterclockwise rotation, whereas poor R-wave progression is commonly observed with clockwise rotation.

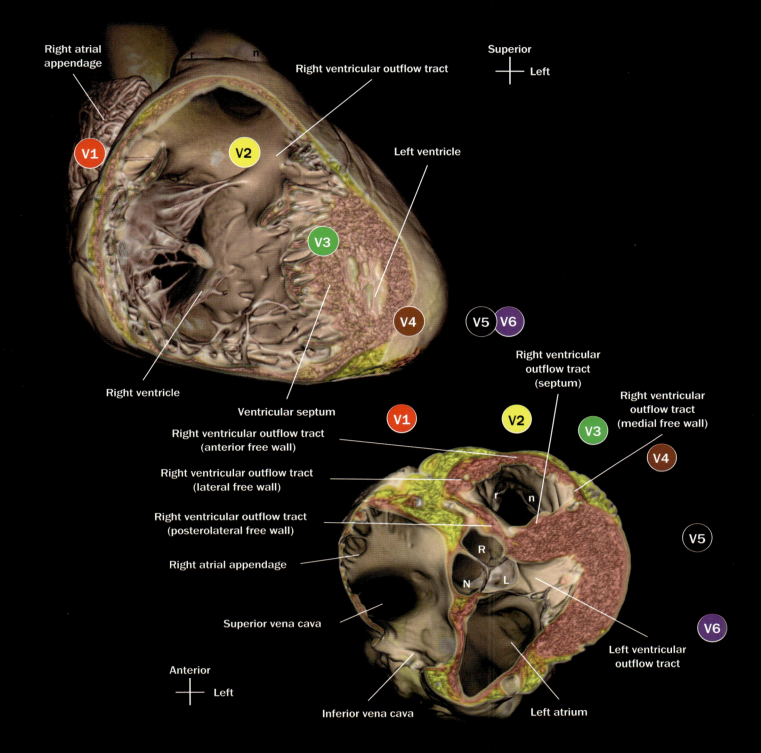

Figure 1-6 Precordial lead location relative to the heart.

In the frontal view, V1 and V2 overlie the right atrial appendage and the right ventricular outflow tract, respectively. Thus, they are often referred to as right-sided precordial leads, which gain insights into pulmonary embolism, right ventricular infarction, Brugada syndrome, and arrhythmogenic right ventricular cardiomyopathy. Caudal view shows why left ventricular hypertrophy shows R-wave progression from V3 to V6. The left ventricular outflow tract exhibits an anterior vector given the posterior orientation relative to the right ventricular outflow tract.

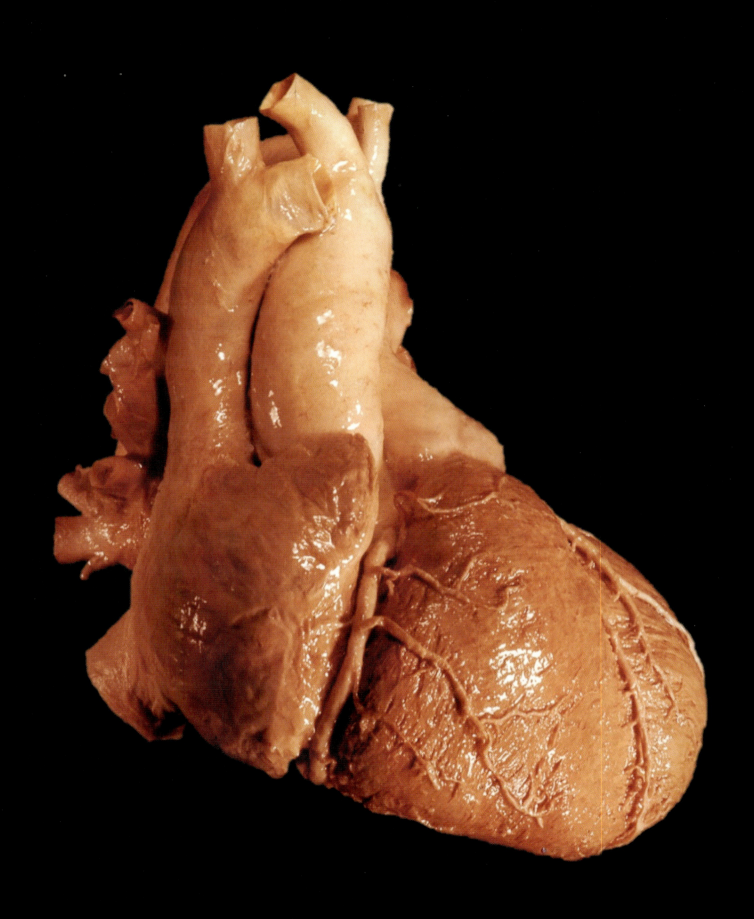

Right Anterior Oblique (RAO) View

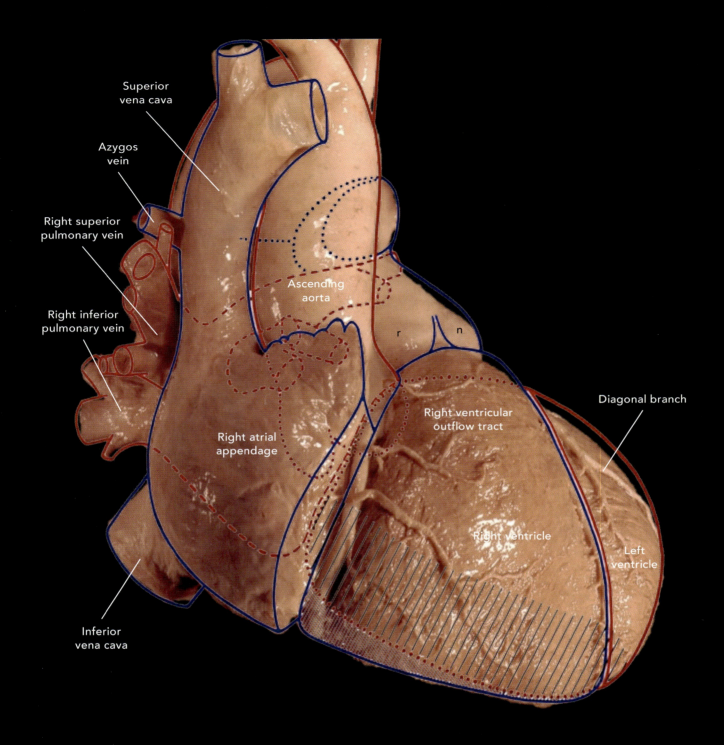

Superior
vena cava

Azygos
vein

Right superior
pulmonary vein

Ascending
aorta

Right inferior
pulmonary vein

r   n

Diagonal branch

Right ventricular
outflow tract

Right atrial
appendage

Right ventricle

Left
ventricle

Inferior
vena cava

Figure 1-7 and Figure 1-8 ▶ Right anterior oblique view.

The right anterior oblique view shows a "side profile" of the heart, allowing for differentiation between the atrium and ventricle. The region of the diagonal branch is the right-hand border of the cardiac silhouette. The pulmonary root is located to the right of and superior to the aortic root.[3] The region behind the high right ventricular outflow tract may not be the ventricular septum, but the proximal anterior interventricular groove involving the left anterior descending artery.

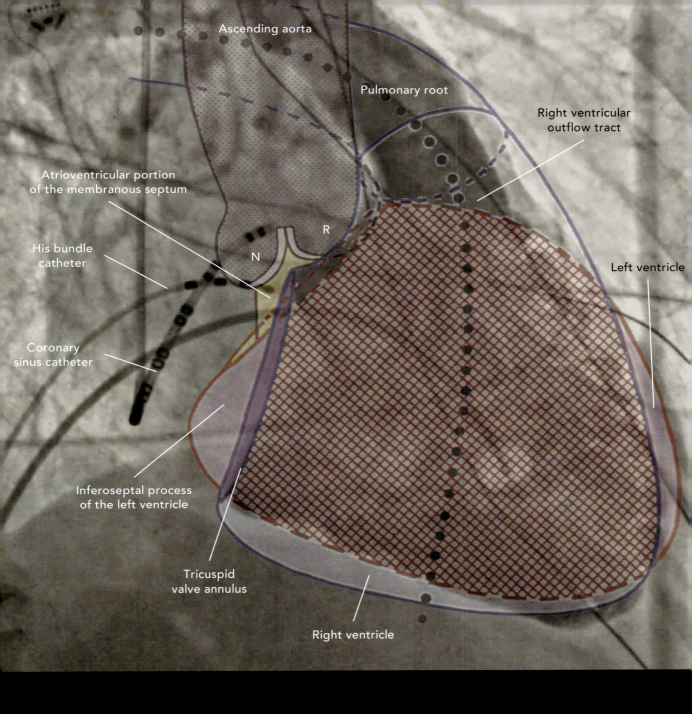

Ascending aorta

Pulmonary root

Right ventricular
outflow tract

Atrioventricular portion
of the membranous septum

R

N

His bundle
catheter

Left ventricle

Coronary
sinus catheter

Inferoseptal process
of the left ventricle

Tricuspid
valve annulus

Right ventricle

An overlay of the chamber over right ventriculography shows that the right ventricle and left ventricle directly overlay one another, except for the most right-hand and left-hand left ventricular borders (pink), the right ventricular outflow tract, and the most inferior right ventricular border (blue). Respecting these boundaries is relevant to avoid potential perforation during intra-right ventricular procedures.[4] His bundle and right ventricular catheters are elongated. In contrast, the coronary sinus catheter is foreshortened a the course is perpendicular to the right anterior oblique plane.

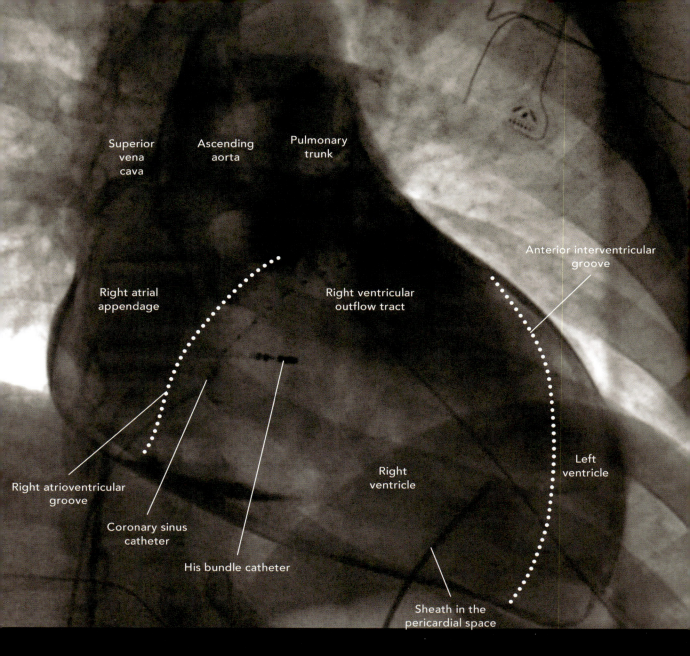

Superior vena cava

Ascending aorta

Pulmonary trunk

Anterior interventricular groove

Right atrial appendage

Right ventricular outflow tract

Right atrioventricular groove

Coronary sinus catheter

His bundle catheter

Right ventricle

Sheath in the pericardial space

Left ventricle

Figure 1-9 ▶ **and Figure 1-10** **Fluoroscopic correlation in the right anterior oblique view.**
The image is created by injection of contrast into the pericardial space. Standard His bundle and coronary sinus catheter positions are shown. The right-hand border of the cardiac silhouette consists of the left ventricle. The left-hand heart border is the right atrial appendage. The right ventricular outflow tract is located to the right of the centrally located aortic root. The right anterior oblique view is the standard view used to insert catheters and pacemaker leads into the right ventricle.

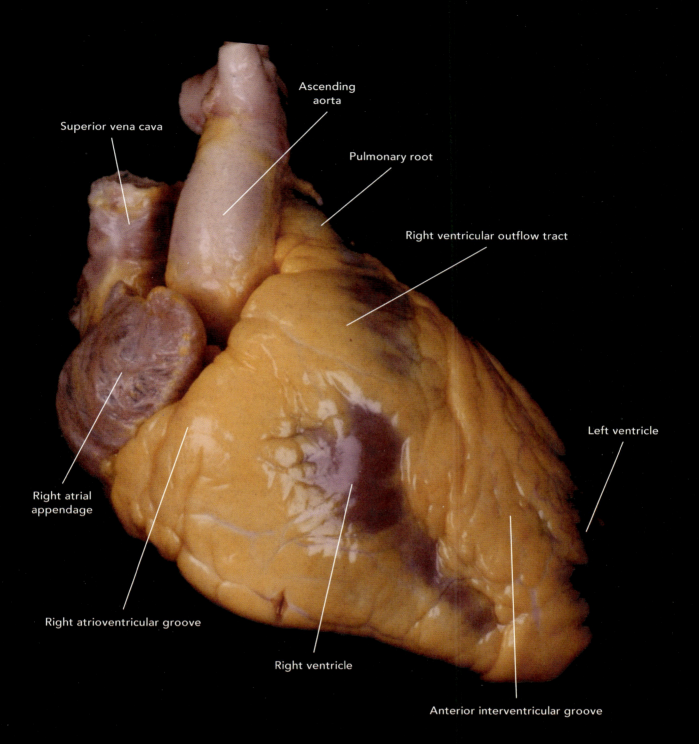

Superior vena cava

Ascending aorta

Pulmonary root

Right ventricular outflow tract

Left ventricle

Right atrial appendage

Right atrioventricular groove

Right ventricle

Anterior interventricular groove

The location of the right atrioventricular junction can often be approximated by the thick epicardial fat of the right atrioventricular groove surrounding the right coronary artery. It is referred to as the radiolucent band on fluoroscopy.[5] Similarly, the coronary sinus orifice location can be estimated on fluoroscopy from the epicardial fat wedging from the inferior crux of the heart toward the central fibrous body. It is the inferior pyramidal space,[6] referred to as the inferior ("posterior") fat pad during fluoroscopy.

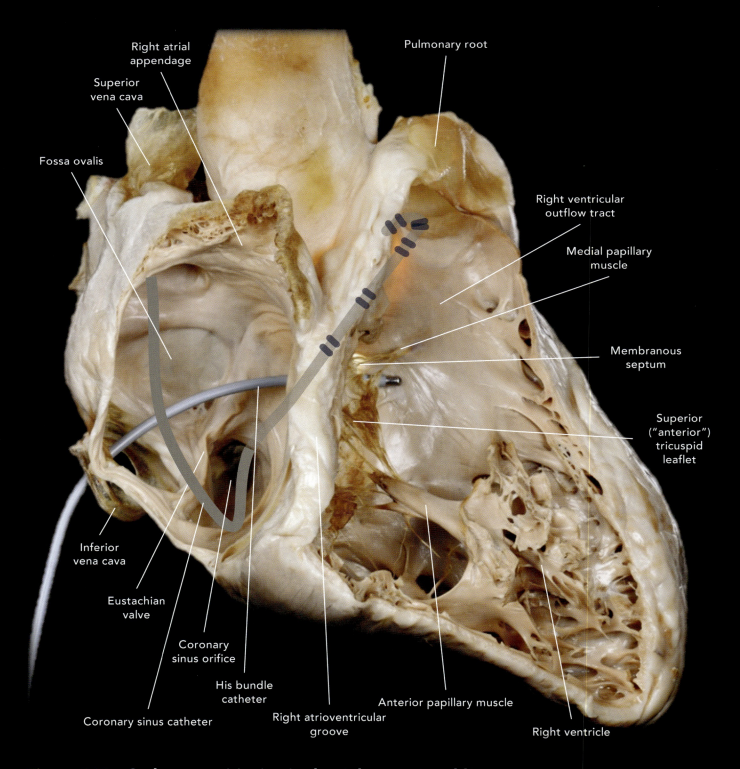

Right atrial appendage

Superior vena cava

Pulmonary root

Fossa ovalis

Right ventricular outflow tract

Medial papillary muscle

Membranous septum

Superior ("anterior") tricuspid leaflet

Inferior vena cava

Eustachian valve

Coronary sinus orifice

His bundle catheter

Coronary sinus catheter

Right atrioventricular groove

Anterior papillary muscle

Right ventricle

Figure 1-11 **Catheter positioning in the right anterior oblique view.**

The coronary sinus catheter represents the divisional plane between the atria and ventricles within the atrioventricular groove. Its proximal part (coronary sinus to proximal great cardiac vein) is generally located on the left atrial side, and its distal side is closer to the ventricular side. Thus, distal electrodes generally record a lower A/V ratio compared to the proximal electrodes with far-field ventricular potential. Importantly, the tricuspid annular plane, demarcated by the right coronary artery, is inferior and apical to the mitral valve annulus.[7]

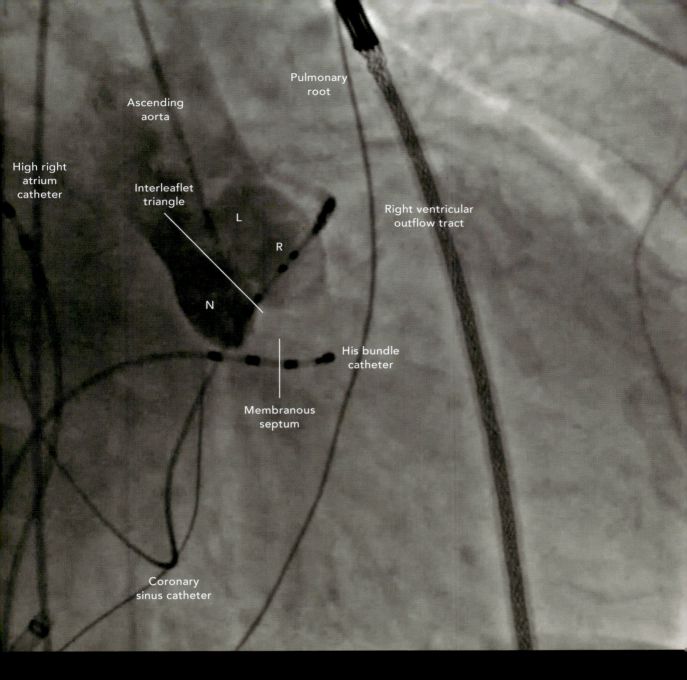

High right
atrium
catheter

Ascending
aorta

Interleaflet
triangle

L

R

N

Pulmonary
root

Right ventricular
outflow tract

His bundle
catheter

Membranous
septum

Coronary
sinus catheter

Figure 1-12 ▶ Aortic root angiography in the right anterior oblique view.

oncoronary and right coronary aortic sinuses are separated. The noncoronary aortic sinus is situated feroposterior to the right and left coronary aortic sinuses. In this view, classical transseptal catheterization as guided by the placement of a pigtail catheter in the noncoronary aortic sinus to avoid aortic puncture the fossa ovalis is generally located on the left side of this sinus. The proximal electrodes of the His undle catheter cross the tricuspid valve annulus adjacent to the interleaflet triangle between the right nd noncoronary aortic sinuses.

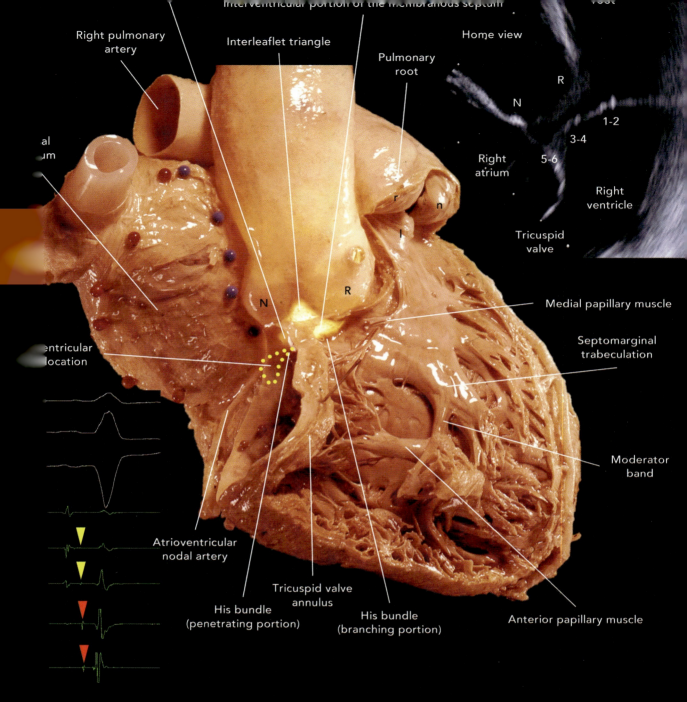

Interventricular portion of the membranous septum

Right pulmonary artery

Interleaflet triangle

Pulmonary root

Home view

R

N

1-2

3-4

5-6

al um

Right atrium

Right ventricle

Tricuspid valve

Medial papillary muscle

N

R

r

n

l

Septomarginal trabeculation

entricular location

Moderator band

Atrioventricular nodal artery

Tricuspid valve annulus

His bundle (penetrating portion)

His bundle (branching portion)

Anterior papillary muscle

1-13 *Spotlight:* Membranous septum and His bundle recording.

...oventricular node lies inferior and basal to the membranous septum. The true His bundle signal (yellow ...ads) is recorded at 5-6, which is at the tricuspid valve annulus, where the ventricular component ...arger than the atrial component. Note that 7-8 records a proximal His bundle signal, where the ...ectrogram is slightly larger than 5-6. The right bundle is recorded on electrodes 3-4 and 1-2 (re... ...ads), which are apical and superior to the His bundle and inferior to the right coronary aortic sinus.

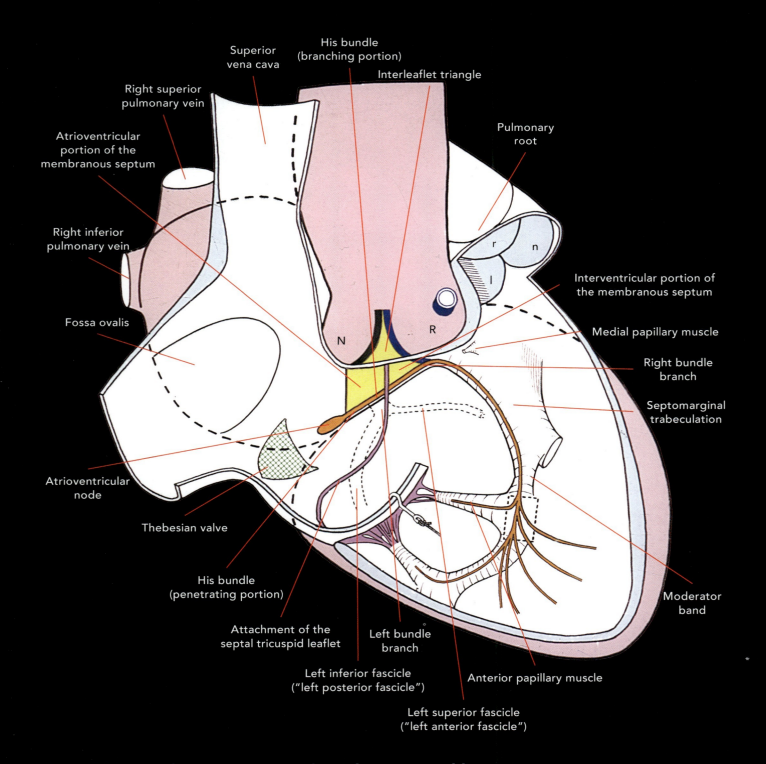

Figure 1-14 **Conduction system in the right anterior oblique view.**

The atrioventricular node is located more inferior and basal to the His bundle. The proximal right bundle branch runs superior and anterior to the left bundle. The membranous septum and the interleaflet triangle (yellow) match the transilluminated specimen (Figure 1-13). The moderator band houses the right bundle branch, which runs from the septum to the free wall of the right ventricle. The thickness, length, and origin of the proximal left bundle branch relative to the membranous septum and septal tricuspid leaflet attachment are variable among individuals.

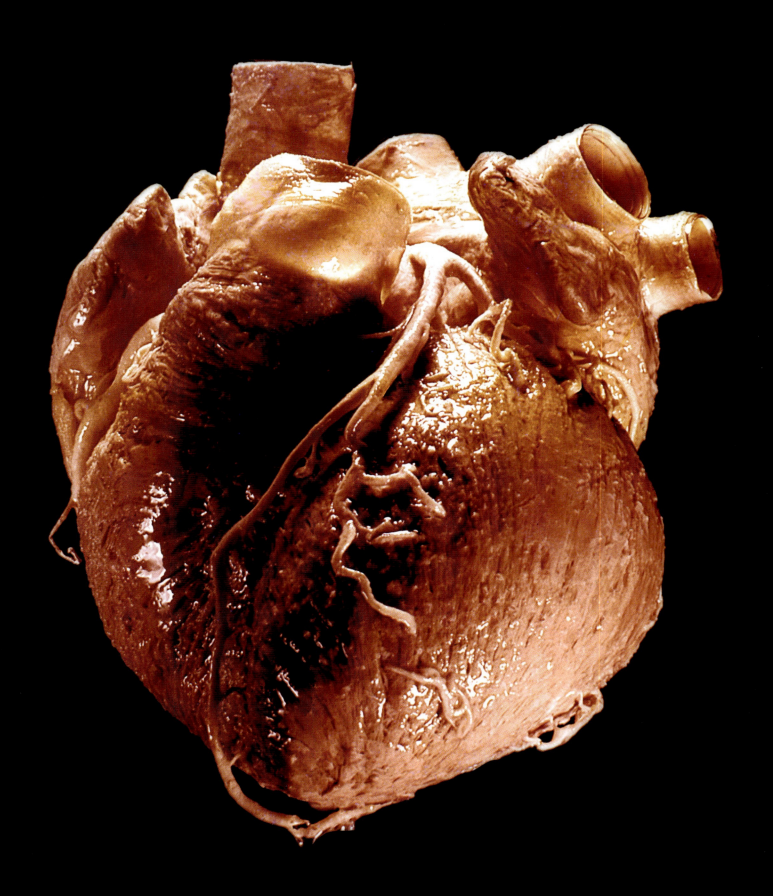

Left Anterior Oblique (LAO) View

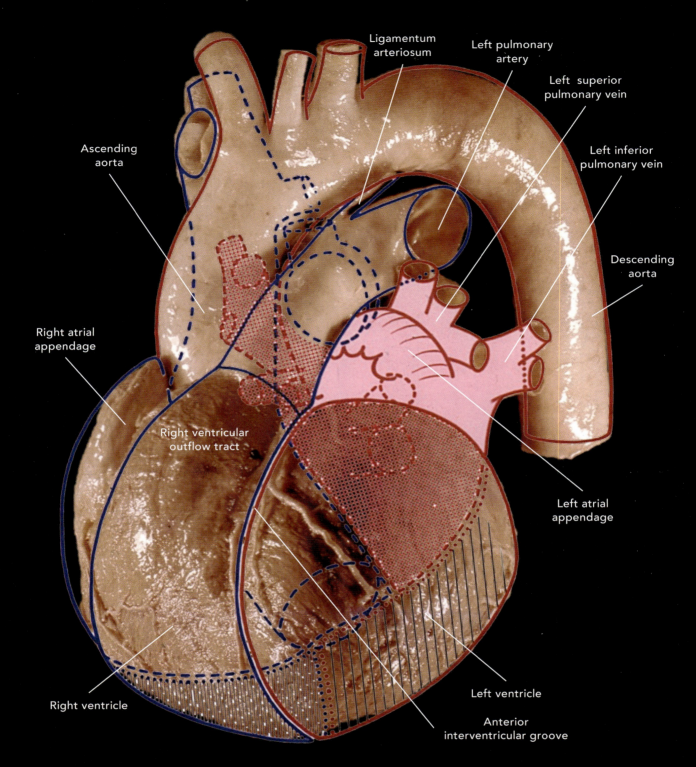

Figure 1-15   Left anterior oblique view.

The right and left ventricles are divided by the anterior interventricular groove. The appropriate left anterior oblique view for a given cardiac orientation is found where the left anterior descending artery runs vertically. Only a small portion of the atria appears behind the ventricular silhouette. The pulmonary veins are foreshortened. The aorta is maximally elongated, which makes this view ideal during the retrograde approach to the left ventricle. The superior vena cava resides behind the ascending aorta. Both arterial trunks are in a crisscross relationship.

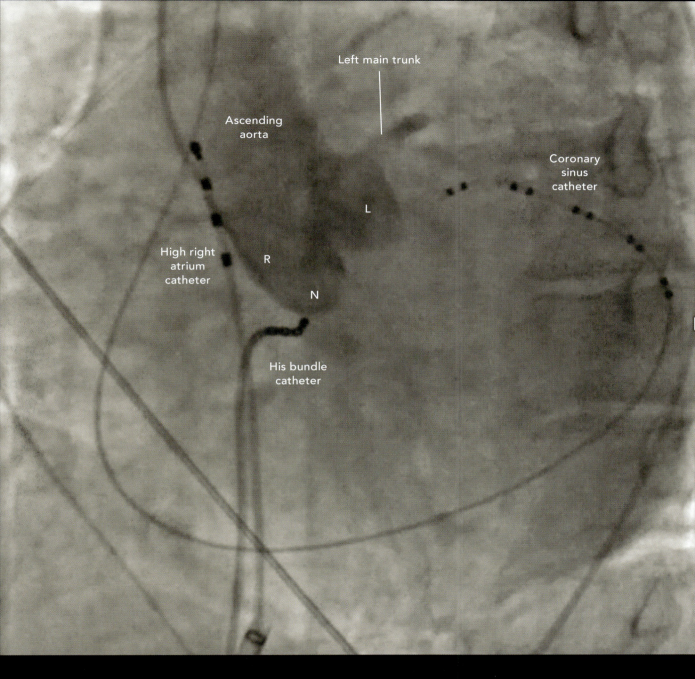

Left main trunk

Ascending
aorta

Coronary
sinus
catheter

L

High right
atrium
catheter

R

N

His bundle
catheter

Figure 1-16 ▶ **Aortic root angiography in the left anterior oblique view.**

The left anterior oblique angulation allows maximal separation of the right and left coronary aortic sinuses in contrast to the right anterior oblique view.[8] The noncoronary aortic sinus is the most inferior one. The left main trunk is visualized from the left coronary aortic sinus. The foreshortened His bundle catheter is immediately adjacent to the noncoronary aortic sinus. The distal coronary sinus catheter approaches the left coronary aortic sinus within the great cardiac vein proximal to the anterior interventricular vein.

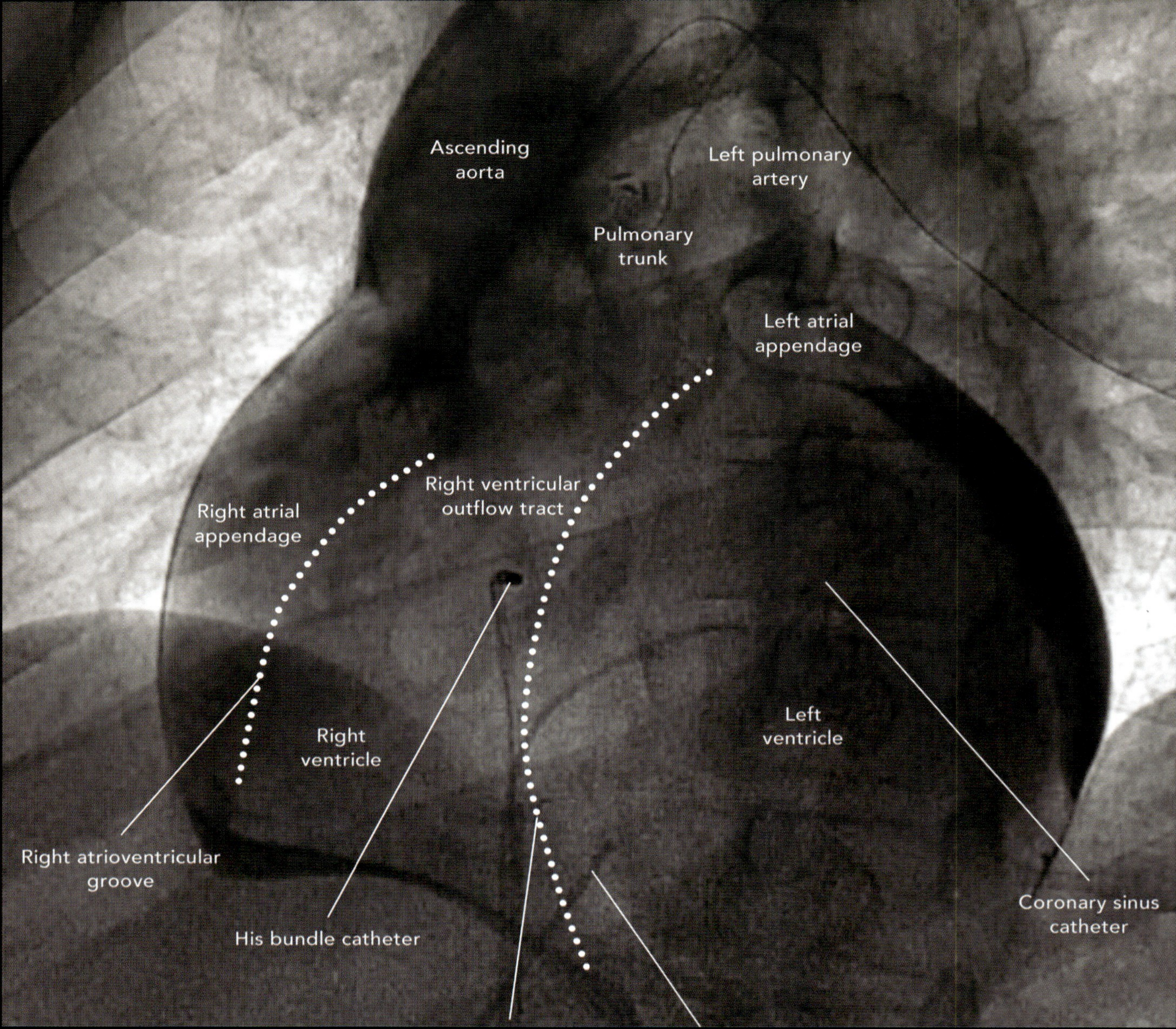
Ascending aorta
Left pulmonary artery
Pulmonary trunk
Left atrial appendage
Right ventricular outflow tract
Right atrial appendage
Right ventricle
Left ventricle
Right atrioventricular groove
His bundle catheter
Coronary sinus catheter

Figure 1-17 and Figure 1-18 Fluoroscopic correlation in the left anterior oblique view.

The image is created by injection of contrast into the pericardial space. Standard His bundle and coronary sinus catheters positions are shown. Only a small apical portion of the atrial appendages can be observed behind each corresponding ventricle. The His bundle catheter is foreshortened, and the coronary sinus catheter is elongated in this view.

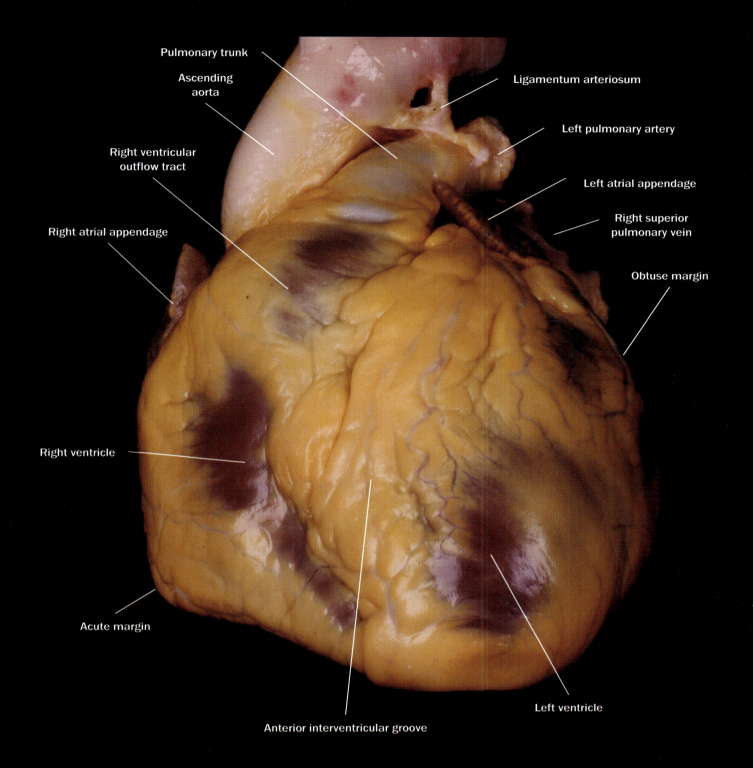

Pulmonary trunk

Ascending aorta

Right ventricular outflow tract

Right atrial appendage

Right ventricle

Acute margin

Ligamentum arteriosum

Left pulmonary artery

Left atrial appendage

Right superior pulmonary vein

Obtuse margin

Left ventricle

Anterior interventricular groove

The left anterior descending artery and the anterior interventricular vein within the thick anterior interventricular groove is in the center, which divides the right and left heart chambers. Thus, this is the classical angiographic view to assess for ventricular septal defects. The anterior wall of the left ventricle is viewed straight on. The right ventricular outflow tract wraps anterosuperior to the left ventricular outflow tract and left anterior to the aortic root.

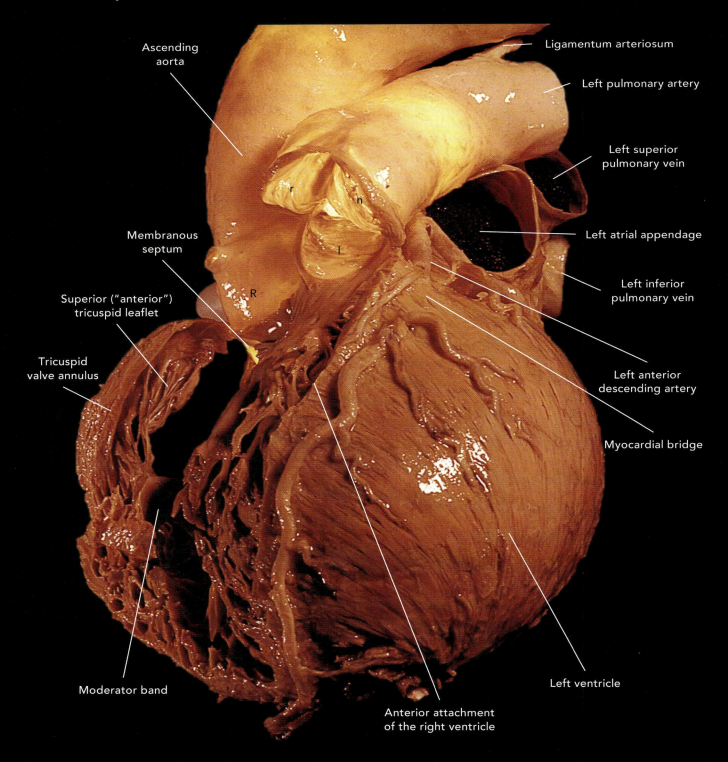

Ascending aorta

Ligamentum arteriosum

Left pulmonary artery

Left superior pulmonary vein

Membranous septum

Left atrial appendage

Left inferior pulmonary vein

Superior ("anterior") tricuspid leaflet

Tricuspid valve annulus

Left anterior descending artery

Myocardial bridge

Moderator band

Left ventricle

Anterior attachment of the right ventricle

Figure 1-19 **Left anterior oblique view with the right ventricle removed.**

The orientations of the intracardiac structures of the right ventricle are evident with the free wall of the right ventricle removed. The transilluminated membranous septum is foreshortened and tilts toward the right anterior and inferior direction along with the aortic root. The anterior attachments of the right ventricle (Figure 3-9) are immediately adjacent to the left anterior descending artery.

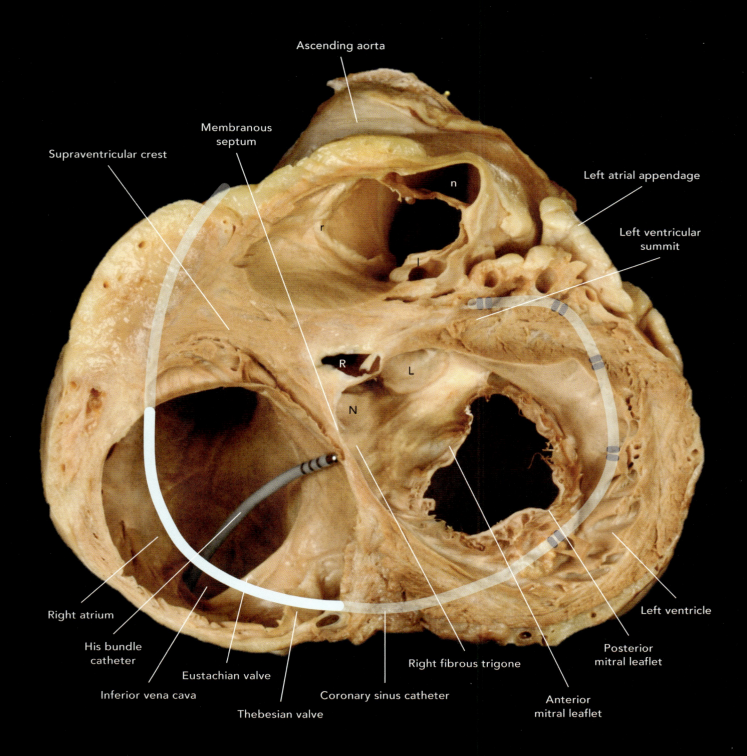

Figure 1-20 Catheter positioning in the left anterior oblique view.

The left anterior oblique view shows the maximally elongated coronary sinus catheter as it enters the coronary sinus orifice and wraps around the left atrioventricular junction within the thick left atrioventricular groove. In general, the distal part of the coronary sinus catheter runs closer to the ventricular side of the mitral annulus compared to more atrialized recordings proximally. The His bundle catheter is foreshortened and placed next to the inferior margin of the membranous septum (Figure 5-6).

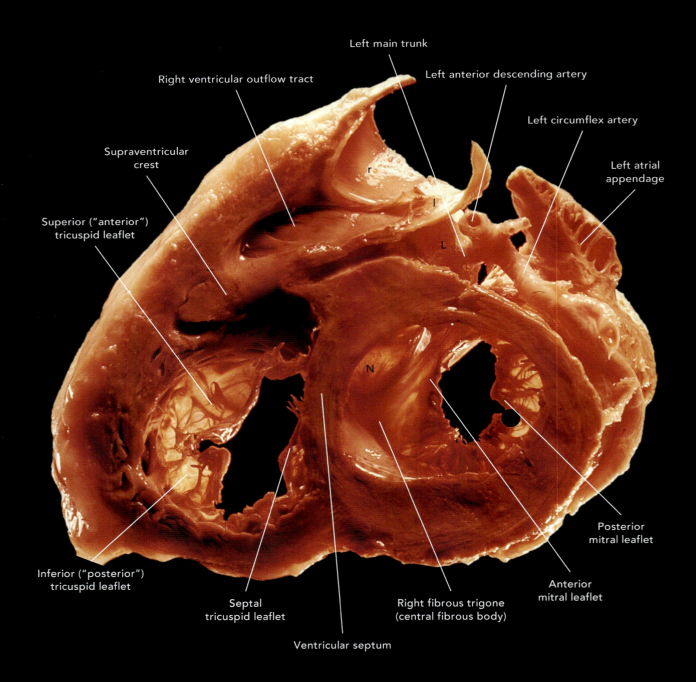

Left main trunk

Right ventricular outflow tract

Left anterior descending artery

Left circumflex artery

Supraventricular crest

Left atrial appendage

Superior ("anterior") tricuspid leaflet

r

I

L

N

Inferior ("posterior") tricuspid leaflet

Posterior mitral leaflet

Septal tricuspid leaflet

Right fibrous trigone (central fibrous body)

Anterior mitral leaflet

Ventricular septum

Figures 1-21 and 1-22   Left anterior oblique sections.

This cross-sectional left anterior oblique section correlates with the standard basal left ventricular short-axis image. The circumflex artery is seen immediately underneath the left atrial appendage, and the proximal left anterior descending artery is adjacent to the left-adjacent pulmonary sinus.

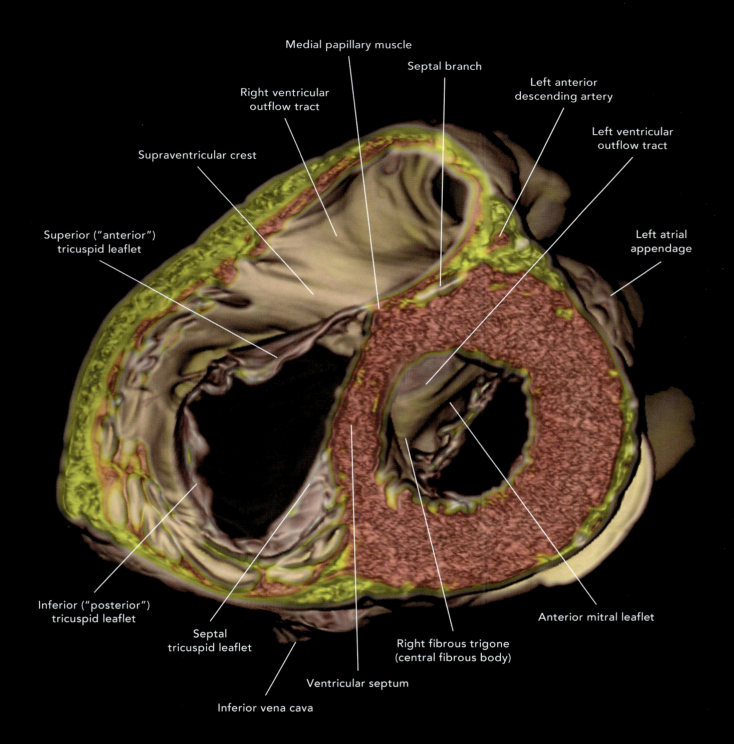

Medial papillary muscle

Septal branch

Left anterior
descending artery

Right ventricular
outflow tract

Left ventricular
outflow tract

Supraventricular crest

Left atrial
appendage

Superior ("anterior")
tricuspid leaflet

Inferior ("posterior")
tricuspid leaflet

Septal
tricuspid leaflet

Anterior mitral leaflet

Right fibrous trigone
(central fibrous body)

Ventricular septum

Inferior vena cava

Note the oblique orientation of the mitral valve orifice[7] and the typical feature of how the chordae tendineae from the medial papillary muscle anchor the superior tricuspid leaflet. The right ventricular outflow tract is located superior to the left ventricular outflow tract.[5] The structure immediately behind the medial portion of the supraventricular crest is the right coronary aortic sinus.

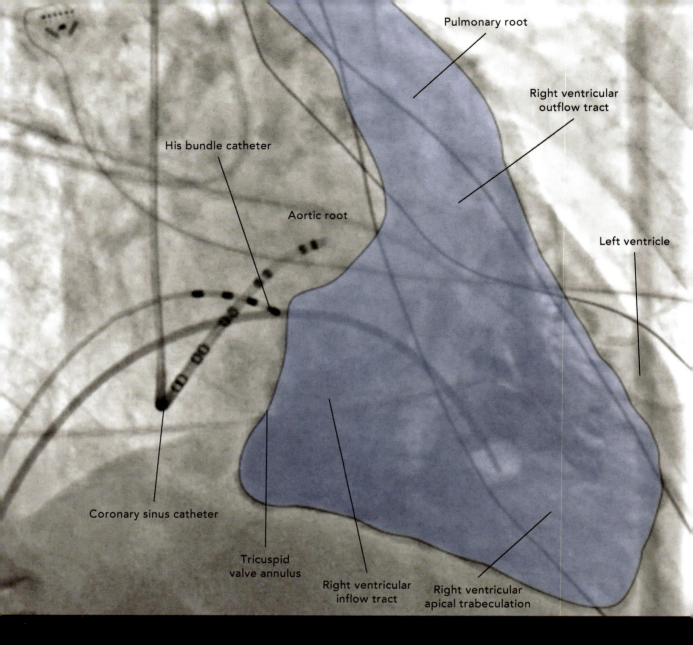

Figure 1-23 ▶ **Right ventricular angiography in the right anterior oblique view.**

Still frame of color-enhanced angiography of the right ventricle to illustrate the borders relative to the right and left anterior oblique views. The left ventricle is the most right-hand border forming the structure in the right anterior oblique view, with the right ventricle within the silhouette.

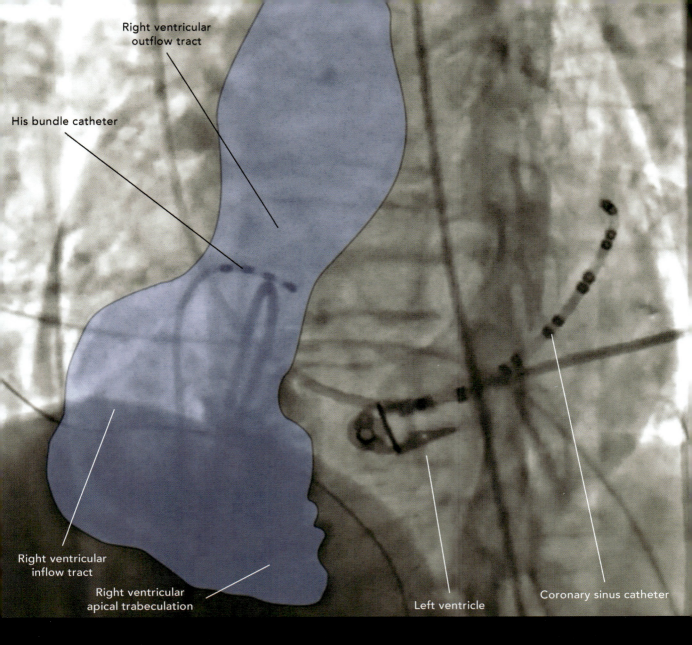

Right ventricular outflow tract

His bundle catheter

Right ventricular inflow tract

Right ventricular apical trabeculation

Left ventricle

Coronary sinus catheter

Figure 1-24 ▶ **Right ventricular angiography in the left anterior oblique view.**

In the left anterior oblique view, the right ventricular outflow tract, pulmonary root, and pulmonary trunk show a crisscross relationship with the left ventricular outflow tract, aortic root, and ascending aorta. Thus, the right ventricular outflow tract is located anterosuperior to the left ventricular outflow tract and left anterior to the aortic root (Figures 1-7, 1-15). The pulmonary root resides left anterosuperior to the aortic root. The pulmonary trunk is located left of the ascending aorta.

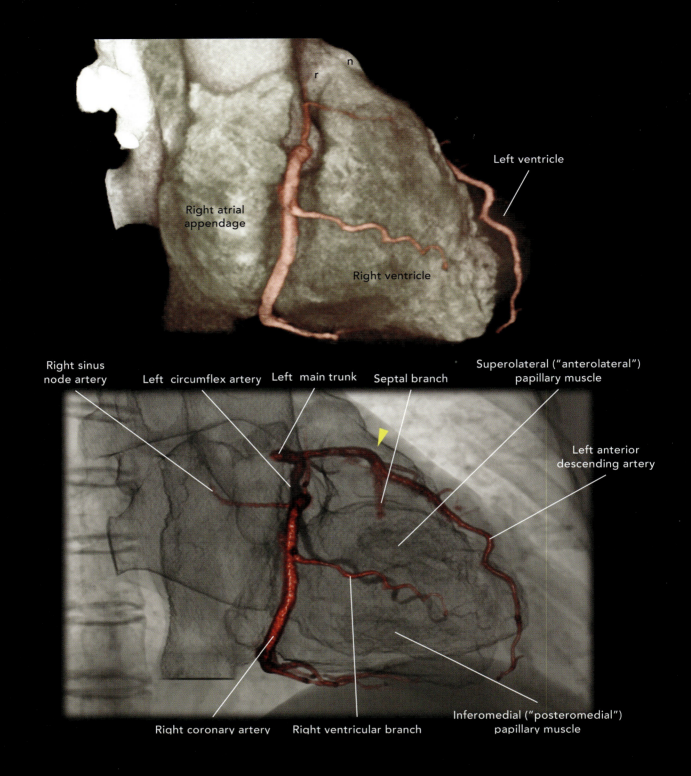

Figure 1-25   Coronary arteries in the right anterior oblique view.

The left anterior descending artery is elongated, with the right coronary artery and left circumflex artery foreshortened. The right sinus node artery is elongated. The diagonal branch demarcates the right-hand border of the contour (Figure 1-7). The relatively horizontal course of the left main trunk and proximal left anterior descending artery skirts the medial wall of the pulmonary root and right ventricular outflow tract, where it creates angulation (yellow arrowhead) to descend vertically and medially relative to the right-hand border of the silhouette.

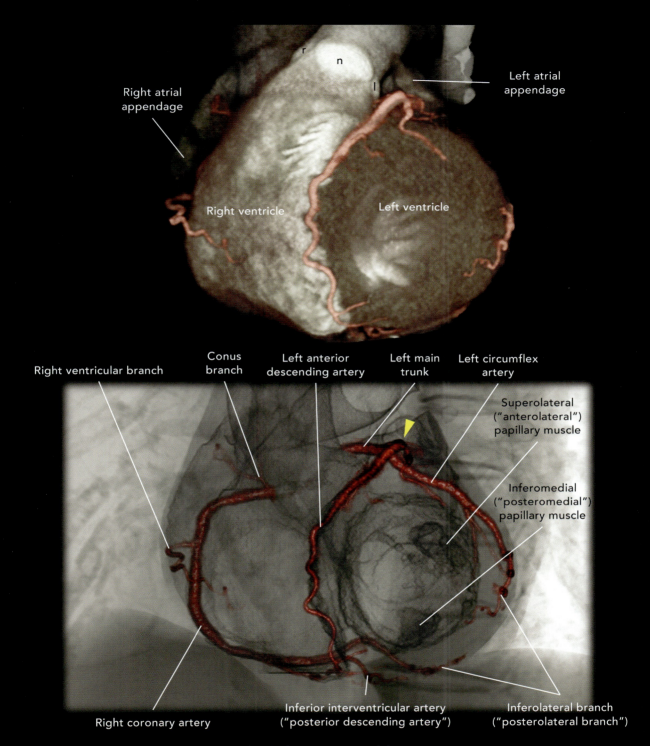

Right atrial appendage

Left atrial appendage

r
n
l

Right ventricle

Left ventricle

Right ventricular branch

Conus branch

Left anterior descending artery

Left main trunk

Left circumflex artery

Superolateral ("anterolateral") papillary muscle

Inferomedial ("posteromedial") papillary muscle

Right coronary artery

Inferior interventricular artery ("posterior descending artery")

Inferolateral branch ("posterolateral branch")

Figure 1-26   Coronary arteries in the left anterior oblique view.

The right coronary artery and the left circumflex artery are fully elongated, and the left anterior descending artery is foreshortened, running directly down the center toward the point of view. The distance from the aortic root to the angulation in the proximal left anterior descending artery (yellow arrowhead) indicates the location of the pulmonary root and distal right ventricular outflow tract wrapped by the artery.

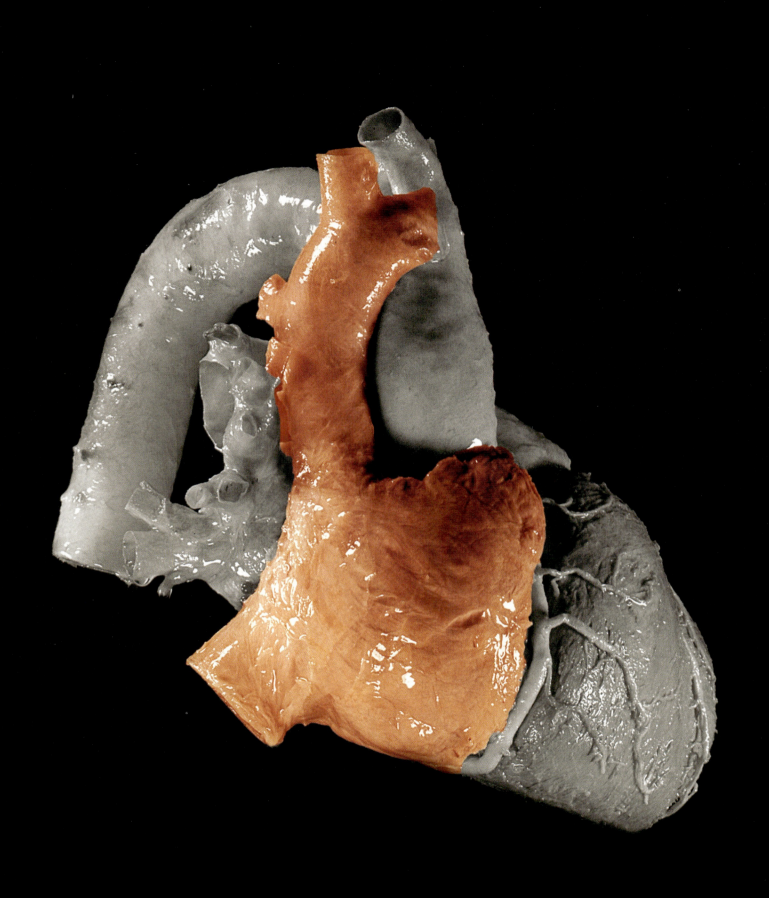

2

The Right Atrium

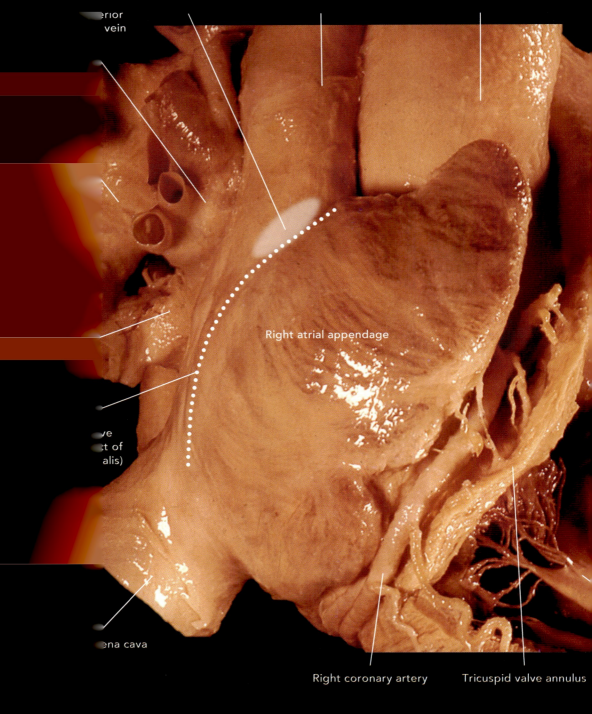

erior
vein

Right atrial appendage

ve
ct of
alis)

ena cava

Right coronary artery   Tricuspid valve annulus

d 2-2   Sinus node.

is a complex that sits at the top of the epicardial and basal side of the ⁻
s) just beneath the level of the right atrial appendage and superior ven

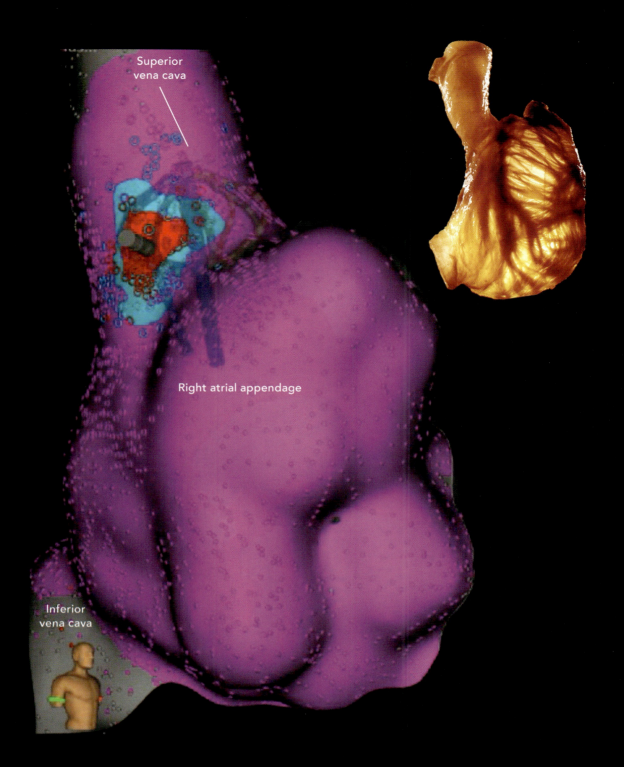

Activation map showing the functional location of the sinus node. Response to isoproterenol typically activates the cells within the superior portions of the sinus node, which makes this aspect the most favorable target during sinus node modification. The right phrenic nerve runs immediately adjacent to the terminal groove or lateral sinus venarum. Displacement of the phrenic nerve using an intrapericardial balloon is an epicardial approach to prevent phrenic nerve injury.[9]

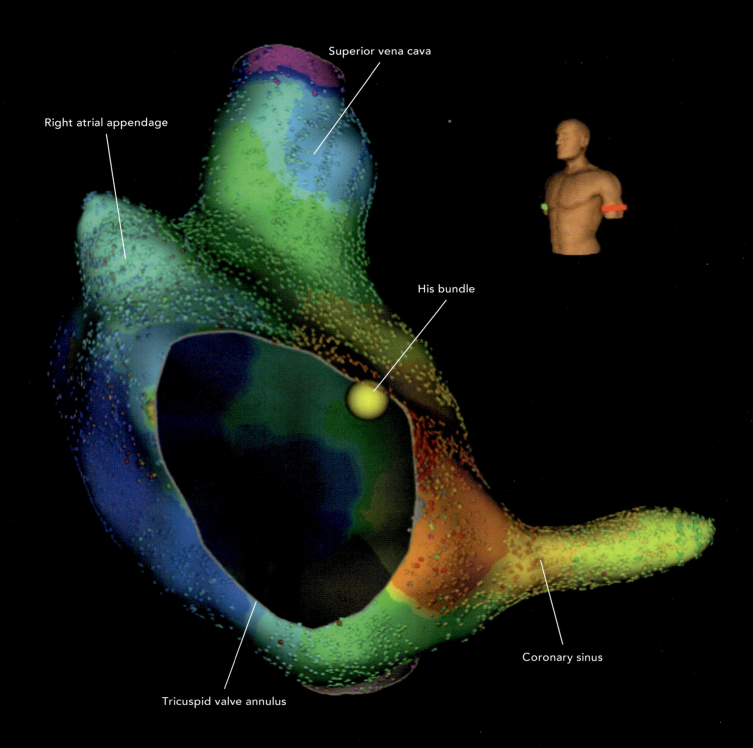

Right atrial appendage

Superior vena cava

His bundle

Coronary sinus

Tricuspid valve annulus

Figures 2-3 and 2-4 Right atrium in the left anterior oblique view.

An electroanatomic map of the right atrium is shown with an identical anatomical image. The clockface of the tricuspid valve annulus is often used to describe the location of atrial tachycardias, accessory pathways, and premature ventricular contractions. The His bundle is typically located between 1:00 to 2:00. The activation map shows earliest retrograde atrial activation in the region of the His bundle, consistent with normal AV nodal fast pathway location.

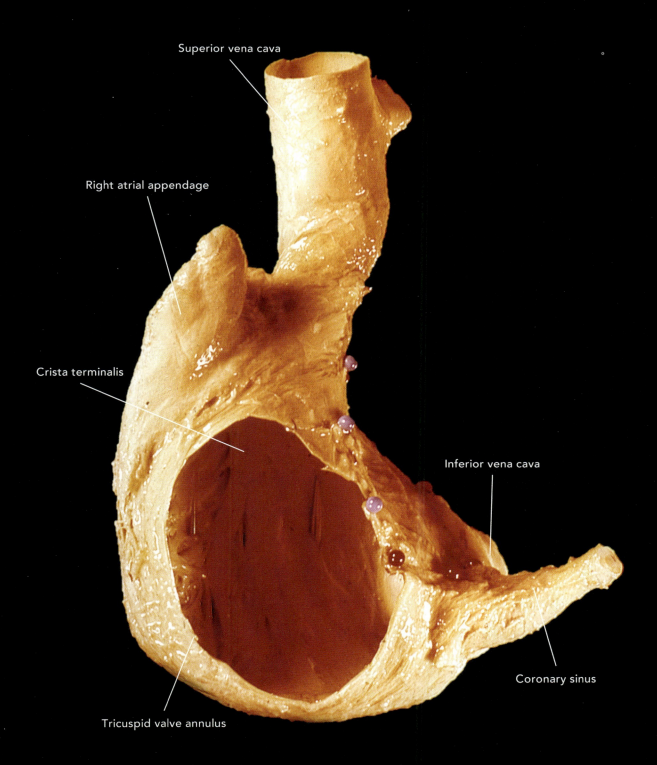

Superior vena cava

Right atrial appendage

Crista terminalis

Inferior vena cava

Coronary sinus

Tricuspid valve annulus

The coronary sinus is typically located between 4:00 to 5:00. The cavotricuspid isthmus is at 6:00. Free-wall arrhythmias are perhaps the most challenging, especially in the region of 8:00 to 10:00, because the operator needs to rotate the catheter counterclockwise and achieve stability, typically requiring a reverse C-shaped catheter profile.

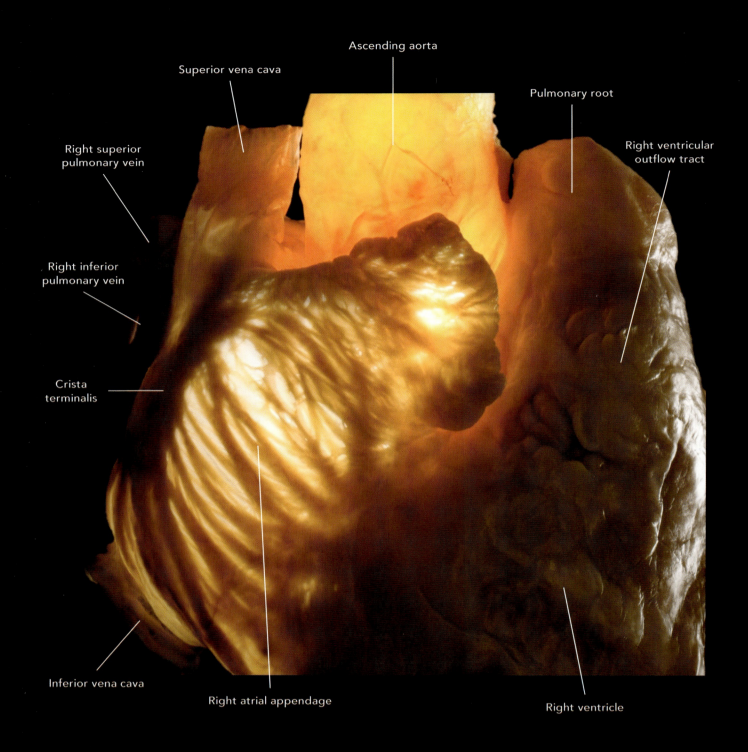

Superior vena cava

Ascending aorta

Pulmonary root

Right superior
pulmonary vein

Right ventricular
outflow tract

Right inferior
pulmonary vein

Crista
terminalis

Inferior vena cava

Right atrial appendage

Right ventricle

Figure 2-5 **External aspect of the crista terminalis in the right anterior oblique view.**

Transilluminated right anterior oblique view of the right atrium showing the crista terminalis demarcating the basal margin of the right atrial appendage. The right atrial appendage consists of multiple pectinate muscles radiating from the crista terminalis toward the right atrial vestibule. Note the thin wall of the right atrial appendage in the region between each pectinate muscle.

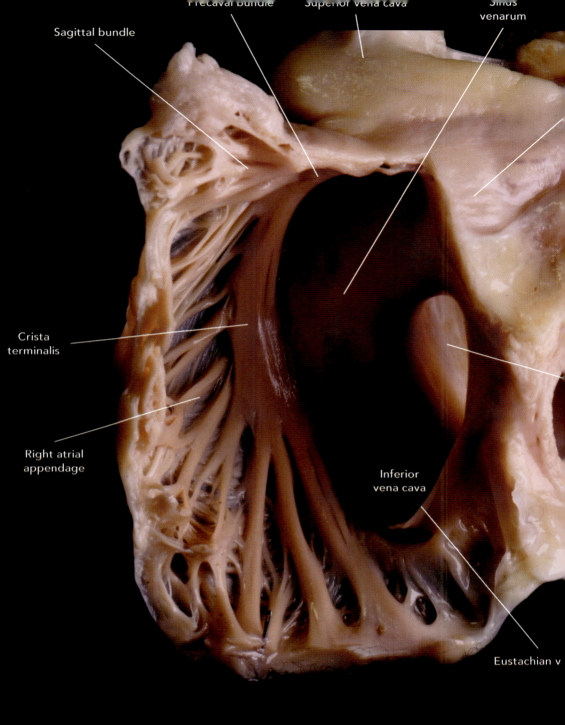

Sagittal bundle

Precaval bundle Superior vena cava Sinus venarum

Crista
terminalis

Right atrial
appendage

Inferior
vena cava

Eustachian v

Figure 2-6 Internal aspect of the crista terminalis in the frontal view.

The crista terminalis demarcates the margin between the right atrial appendage, with

muscles, and the sinus venarum, with a smooth endocardial surface. The pectinate

uperior, lateral, and inferior part of the right atrium, including the cavotricuspid isthm

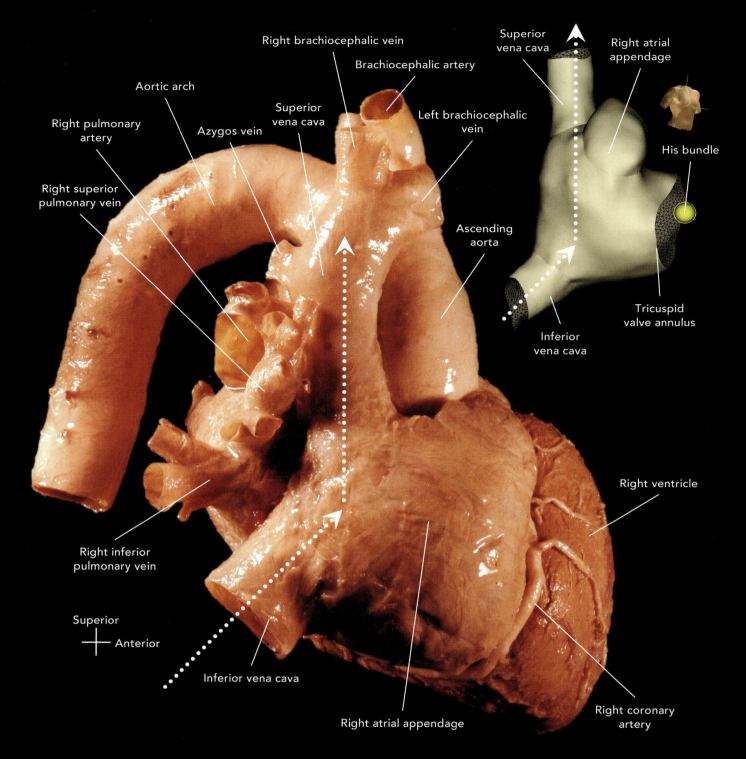

Figure 2-7 Bicaval relationship in the right lateral view.

The axis of the inferior vena cava creates an obtuse angle with the vertical axis of the superior vena cava. The smaller the angle, the more anterior the bias for catheters placed from the inferior approach. This can often challenge transseptal puncture, making it necessary and more difficult to rotate the needle clockwise toward the fossa ovalis to avoid aortic puncture. Recognition of this nonlinear caval relationship is important, and a posterior tilt upon entry into the right atrium can reduce the risk for right atrial appendage perforation.

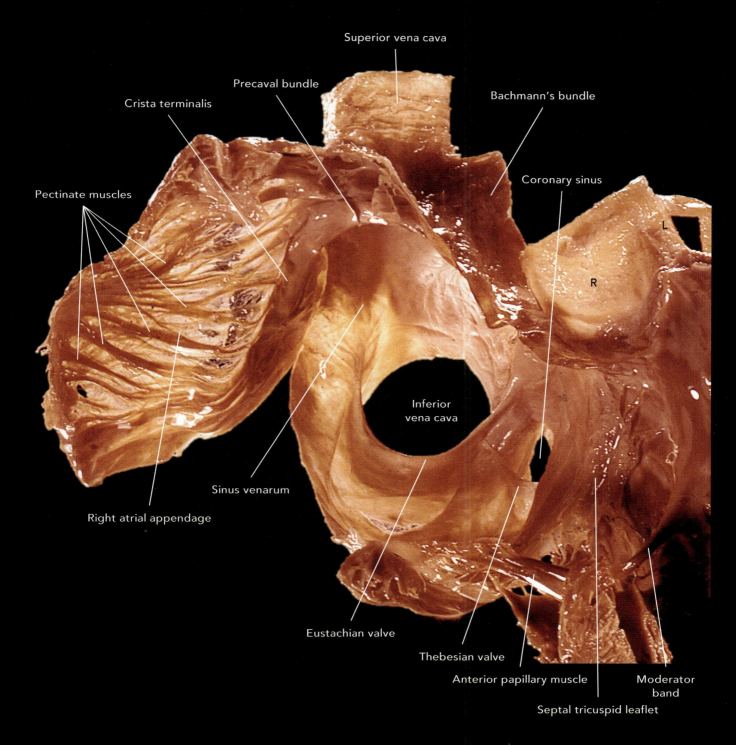

Figure 2-8 **Right atrium through a longitudinal section down the crista terminalis.**

In this frontal view, the orifice of the inferior vena cava appears en face, in contrast to that of the superior vena cava. The right atrium is incised along the crista terminalis, revealing the thin nature of the right atrial free wall with multiple pectinate muscles. Upon entry into the right atrium, the Eustachian valve appears as a semicircular obstacle that attaches to the septum along the anterior limbus of the fossa ovalis. In cases with a prominent Eustachian valve, cannulation to the coronary sinus from the femoral approach can be challenging.

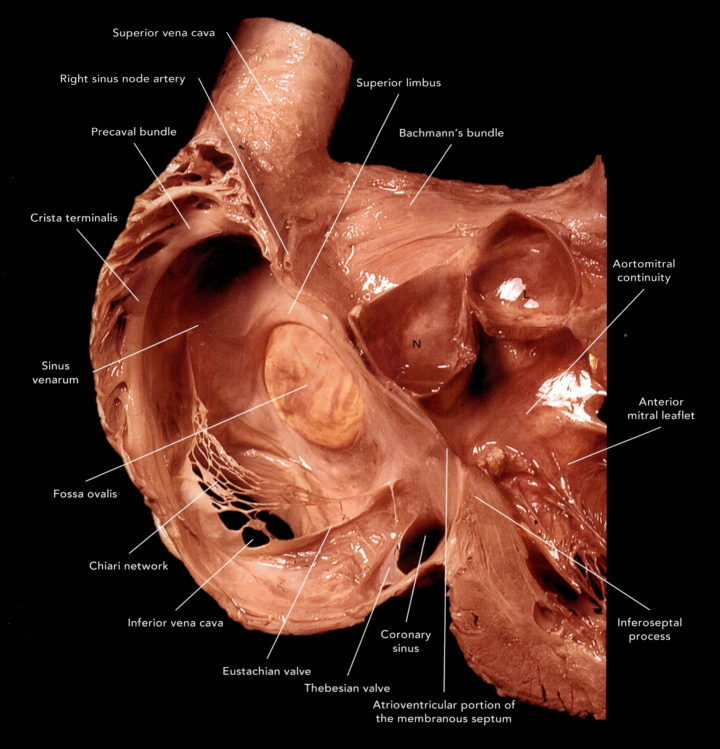

Figure 2-9 **Fossa ovalis in the frontal view.**

The atrial septum, including the floor of the fossa ovalis (primary septum), tilts toward the right anterior and inferior direction. Therefore, even though both the superior and inferior vena cavae are the septal side structures, the inferior vena cava orifice is located medial to the superior vena cava orifice. Thus, an atrial transseptal puncture is far easier from the inferior approach than from the superior approach. This tilting angle of the fossa ovalis shows wide individual variation and is affected by the tilting angle of the ascending aorta. Note the prominent Chiari network.

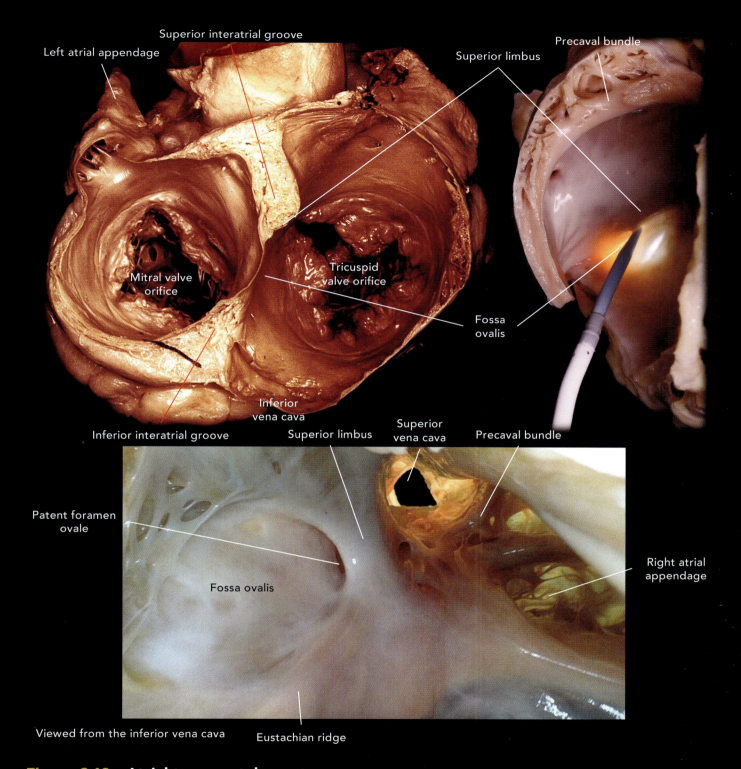

Figure 2-10 **Atrial transseptal puncture.**

With lipomatous hypertrophy, the superior limbus can be prominent (upper left). The superior limbus is a bank between the superior vena cava and the fossa ovalis. The floor of the fossa ovalis tilts toward the right atrium, covering the medial orifice of the inferior vena cava. Thus, when viewed from the inferior vena cava orifice (bottom), the fossa ovalis looks like a medial-side roof. When the system is pulled back across the superior limbus, a typical jump-in motion of the system can be observed, the classical sign to confirm the location of the fossa ovalis (upper right).

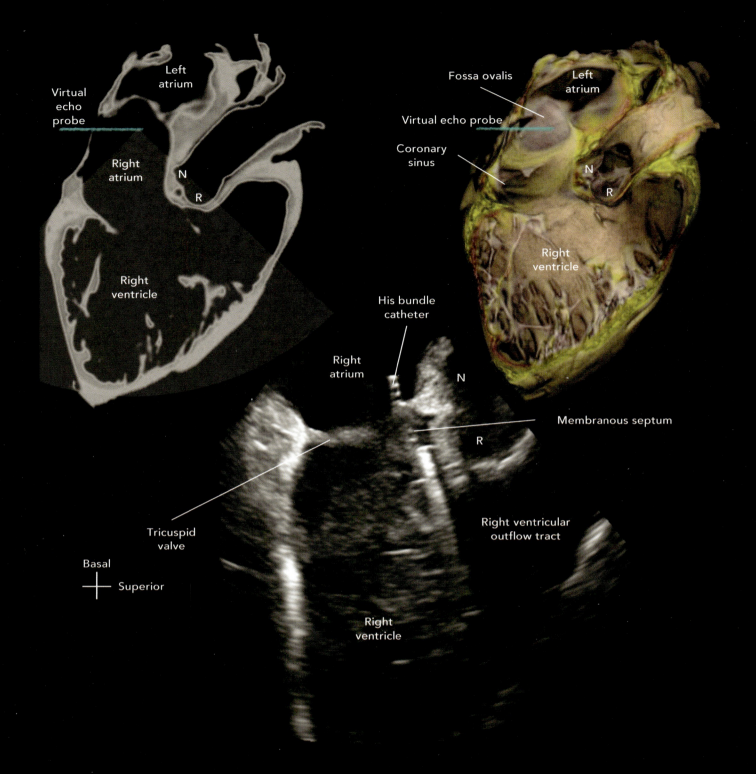

Figure 2-11 **Home view on intracardiac echocardiography.**

The "home view" of intracardiac echocardiography is achieved with a vertical and straight orientation of the probe within the right atrium. In this position, the probe looks through the tricuspid valve into the right ventricle, with a section of the aortic root that lies posterior to the right ventricular outflow tract. The home view in situ is typically visualized at 90 degrees, rotated clockwise relative to the intrinsic orientation of the heart.[10] This home view corresponds to the right anterior oblique sections of the right heart.

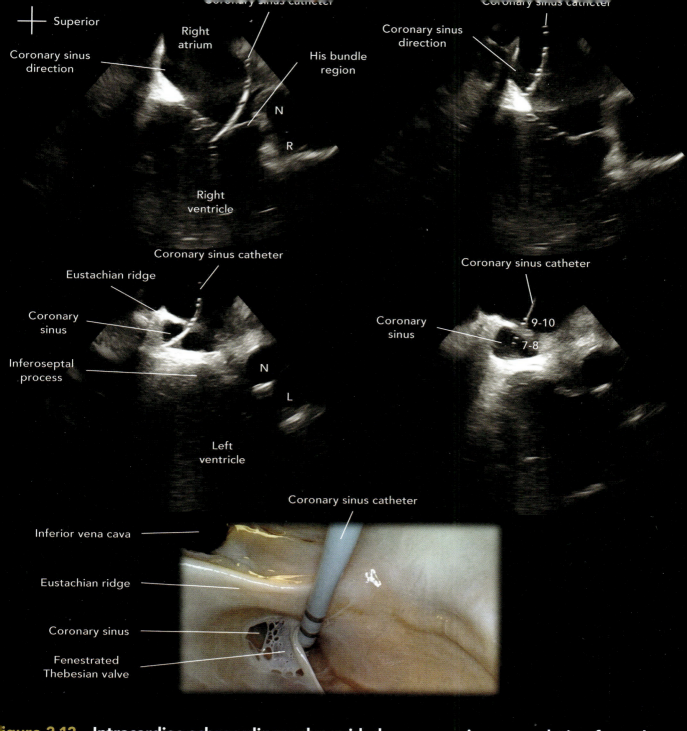

Figure 2-12   Intracardiac echocardiography-guided coronary sinus cannulation from the femoral approach.

A decapolar catheter is withdrawn from the His bundle region (upper left). The catheter is deflected toward the inferior tricuspid valve annulus (upper right). The intracardiac echocardiography probe then is slightly torqued clockwise to expose the coronary sinus orifice. With slight clockwise torque and advancement the catheter jumps into the coronary sinus (middle left), with visualization of the proximal electrodes 9-10 at the level of the orifice (middle right). The bottom panel is the corresponding endoscopic image.

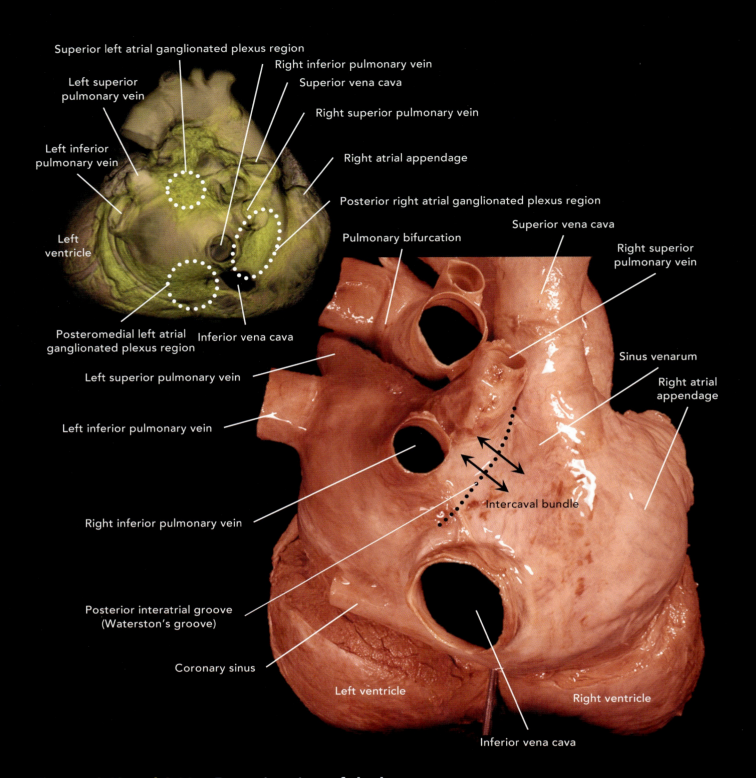

Figures 2-13 and 2-14   Posterior view of the heart.

This posterior view highlights the nonlinear bicaval relationship and medial location of the inferior vena cava relative to the superior vena cava. The nondescript demarcation between the two chambers consists of the posterior interatrial groove, also referred to as the Waterston's groove, which is incised for surgical access to the left atrium. This region between the two atria has also significant anatomical relevance for cardioneuroablation as the posterior right atrial ganglionated plexus region lies within the epicardial fat within the Waterston's groove.[11]

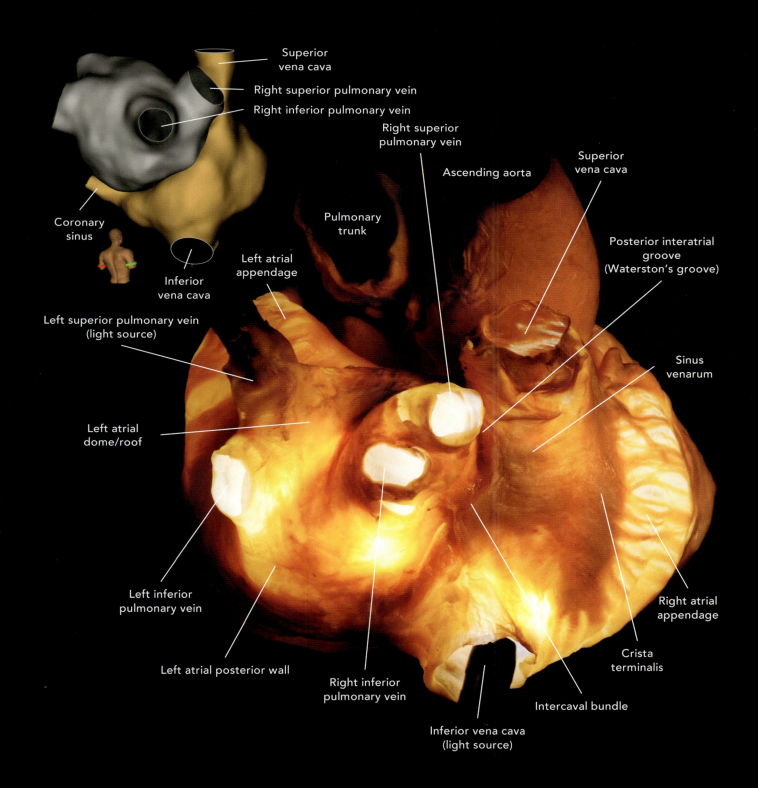

Superior
vena cava

Right superior pulmonary vein

Right inferior pulmonary vein

Coronary
sinus

Inferior
vena cava

Left superior pulmonary vein
(light source)

Left atrial
dome/roof

Left inferior
pulmonary vein

Left atrial posterior wall

Right superior
pulmonary vein

Ascending aorta

Pulmonary
trunk

Left atrial
appendage

Superior
vena cava

Posterior interatrial
groove
(Waterston's groove)

Sinus
venarum

Right atrial
appendage

Crista
terminalis

Intercaval bundle

Right inferior
pulmonary vein

Inferior vena cava
(light source)

The anterior portion of the right superior pulmonary vein lies adjacent to the posterior aspect of the superior vena cava at the posterior interatrial groove. During pulmonary vein isolation, far-field superior vena cava activity may require differential pacing to confirm an entrance block into the antrum of the right superior pulmonary vein. The intercaval bundles are important interatrial connections that may confound the ability to achieve isolation of the right-sided veins in the absence of ablation within the carina.

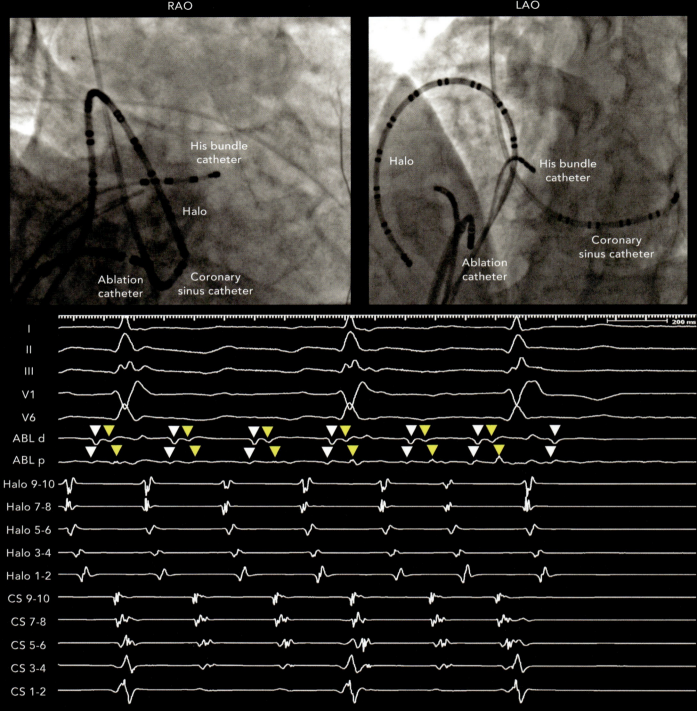

RAO

LAO

His bundle catheter

Halo

Ablation catheter

Coronary sinus catheter

Halo

His bundle catheter

Ablation catheter

Coronary sinus catheter

Figure 2-15 *Spotlight:* Common typical (counterclockwise) atrial flutter.

A halo linear catheter in the right atrium with proximal and distal electrodes on the atrial septum and low lateral wall, respectively, allows for rapid diagnosis of flutter directionality. Coronary sinus activation is typically proximal to distal in common atrial flutter with a circuit around the tricuspid valve annulus. Termination of flutter is observed between low lateral right atrial activation and the proximal coronary sinus with the creation of isthmus block. Splitting of local potentials (arrowheads) is observed on the ablation catheter prior to termination of flutter.

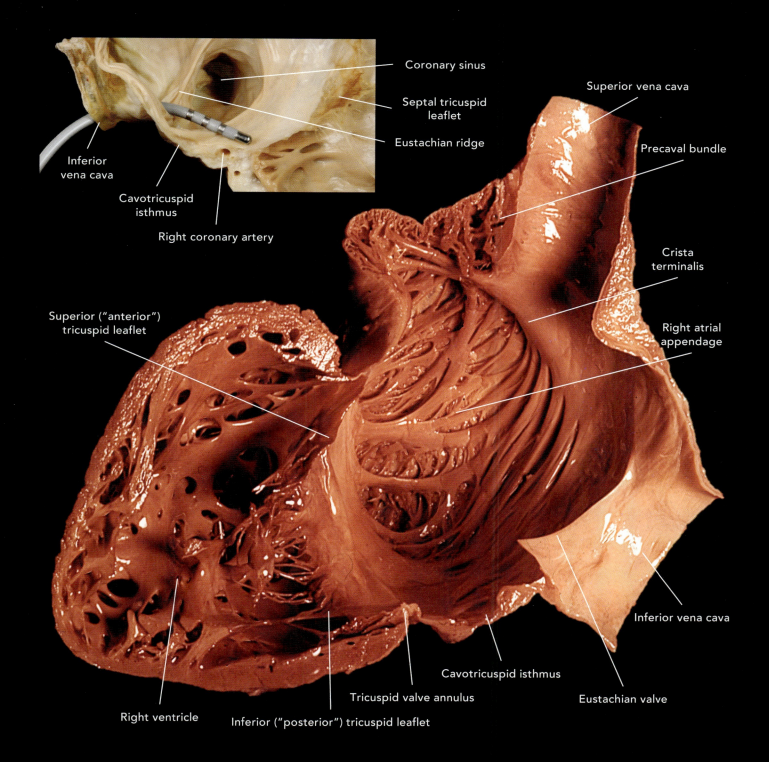

Figure 2-16 Left lateral view of the cavotricuspid isthmus.

The topography of the cavotricuspid isthmus is highly variable, with some areas being relatively flat and others having prominent pouches and trabeculations. The medial aspect tends to have more pouches adjacent to the orifice of the coronary sinus, whereas the lateral aspect may have more ridges and trabeculations. In this regard, the use of intracardiac echocardiography may guide the most optimal catheter profile, as the irregularity of the endocardial surface and height of the Eustachian valve are difficult to assess based on fluoroscopy alone.

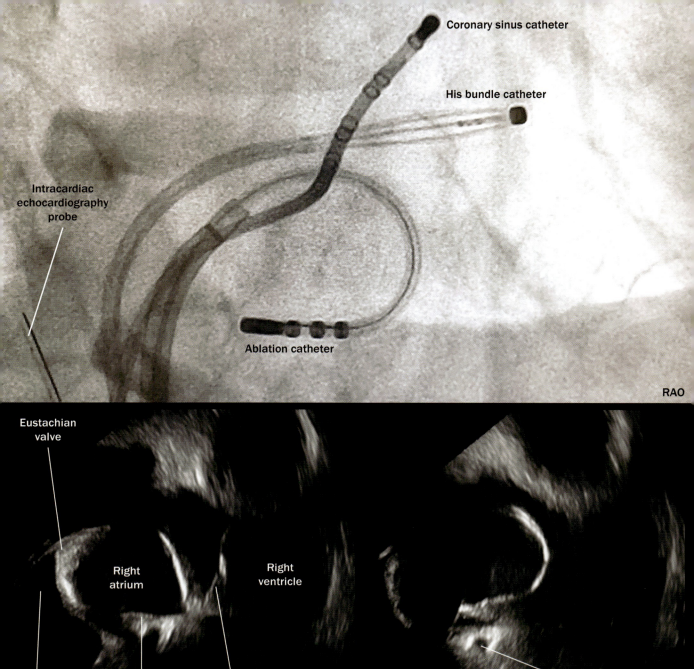

Figure 2-17 ▶ **and Figure 2-18**   **Prolapsed catheter profile for typical flutter ablation.**

Home view on intracardiac echocardiography shows two catheter profiles to achieve cavotricuspid isthmus ablation. With a prominent Eustachian valve, tissue contact is limited by the top of the fulcrum when dragging an ablation catheter back from the tricuspid valve annulus. In such cases, the ablation catheter should be prolapsed with a large curl, with the aid of a steerable sheath for inferior deflection.

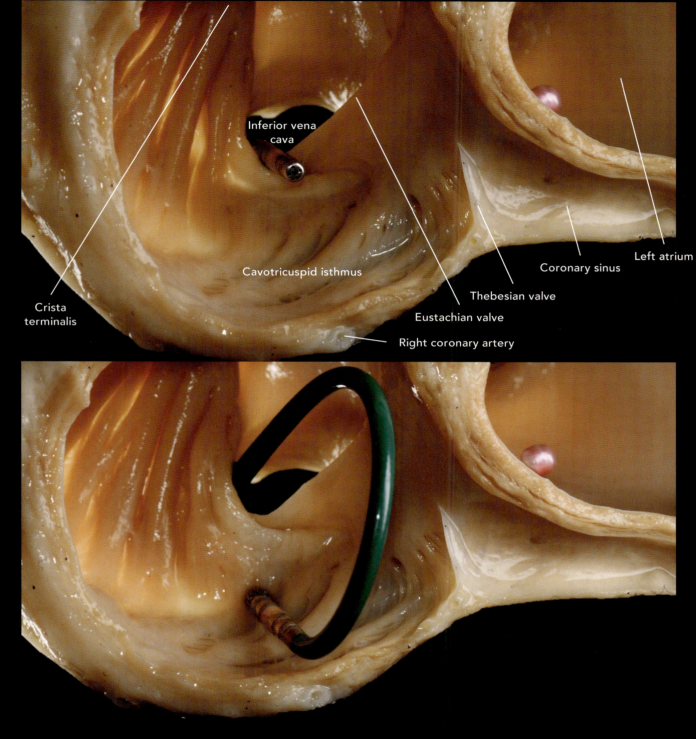

Inferior vena cava

Cavotricuspid isthmus

Crista terminalis

Coronary sinus

Left atrium

Thebesian valve

Eustachian valve

Right coronary artery

With this approach, the catheter is undeflected to achieve contact with the tissue. The proximity of the right coronary artery[12] is important to note during ablation of the cavotricuspid isthmus, as injury and infarction have been reported.[13] The presence of epicardial fat, seen with increased echogenicity, and coronary flow are fortuitous barriers to effective ablation of the artery.

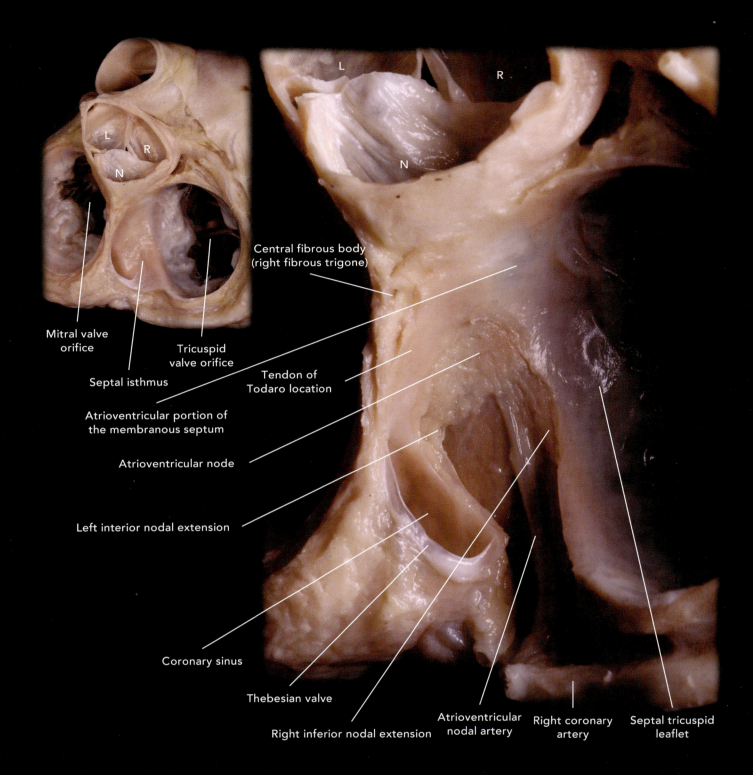

Central fibrous body
(right fibrous trigone)

Mitral valve
orifice

Tricuspid
valve orifice

Septal isthmus

Tendon of
Todaro location

Atrioventricular portion of
the membranous septum

Atrioventricular node

Left interior nodal extension

Coronary sinus

Thebesian valve

Atrioventricular
nodal artery

Right coronary
artery

Septal tricuspid
leaflet

Right inferior nodal extension

Figure 2-19   Triangle of Koch.

The boundaries of the triangle of Koch are 1) the coronary sinus orifice, 2) the septal tricuspid leaflet attachment, and 3) and the tendon of Todaro. The tendon of Todaro is a subendocardial thin fiber strand extending from the Eustachian valve toward the central fibrous body. Removal of the right atrial wall at the floor of the triangle of Koch with epicardial fat wedging from the inferior crux toward the central fibrous body, the inferior pyramidal space,[14] exposes the atrioventricular node and its feeding artery within the triangle. Thus, they are epicardial structures.

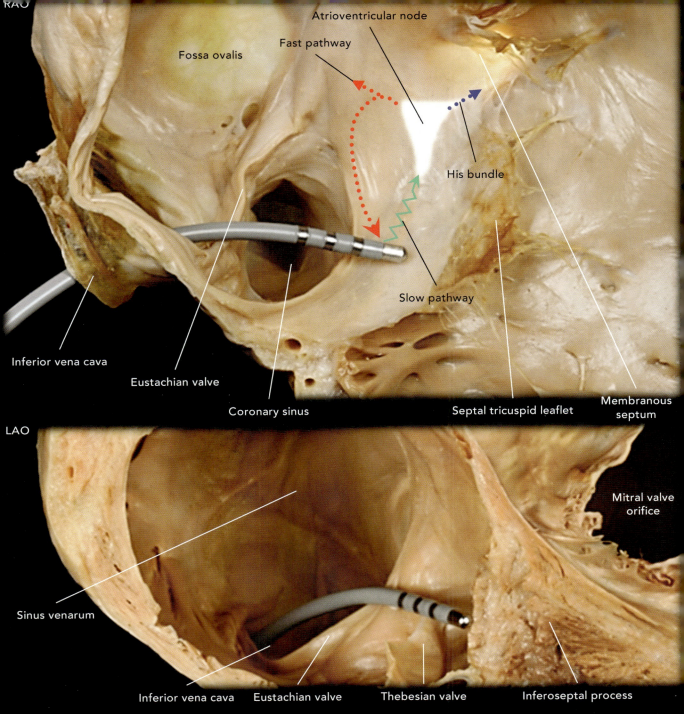

Figure 2-20 *Spotlight:* **Atrioventricular nodal reentrant tachycardia.**

The triangle of Koch is not a flat plane, but a curved structure with an apical and medial floor (Figure 2-29). The slow pathway location lies immediately anterior to the coronary sinus orifice, with the most optimal A/V ratio of 1:3-4, preferencing the ventricular side of the right atrial vestibule at the septal isthmus between the coronary sinus orifice and tricuspid valve annulus. The atrioventricular node is located inferior and posterior to the membranous septum. Ablation at or above the level of the roof of the coronary sinus increases the risk of damage to the fast pathway fibers of the atrioventricular nodal region.

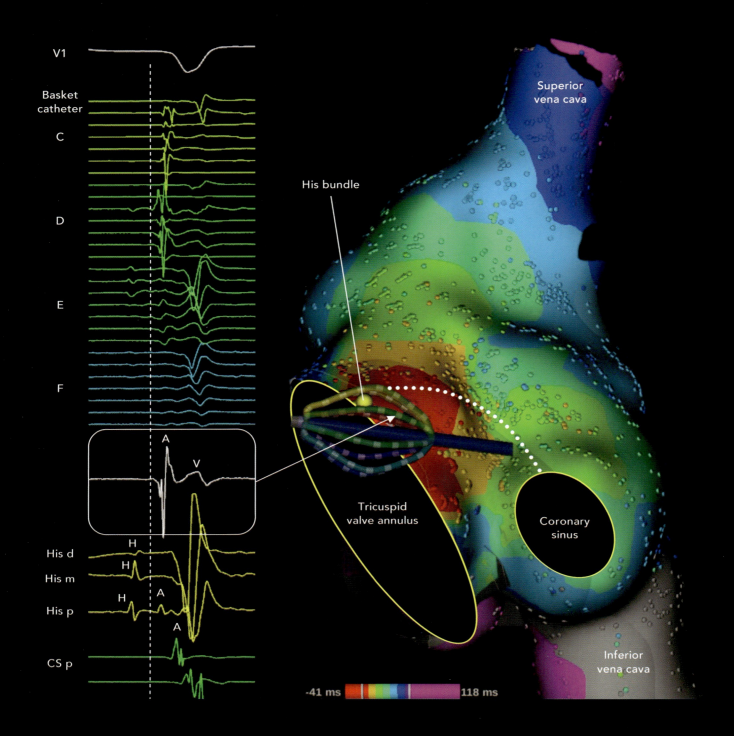

Figures 2-21 and 2-22 **Location of the fast and slow pathways with high-resolution mapping.**

The traditional region of the earliest atrial activation of the retrograde fast pathway during common atrioventricular nodal reentrant tachycardia in the right atrium is immediately posterior to the His bundle. Eccentric left atrial inputs have been described as left-sided slow pathway near the coronary sinus roof (Figure 4-7) in rare cases. The superior ("anterior"), mid, and inferior ("posterior") regions of the septum are also used to classify accessory pathway locations (Figure 2-23). These subtle anatomic differences can result in significant changes in the electrocardiographic axis and morphology.

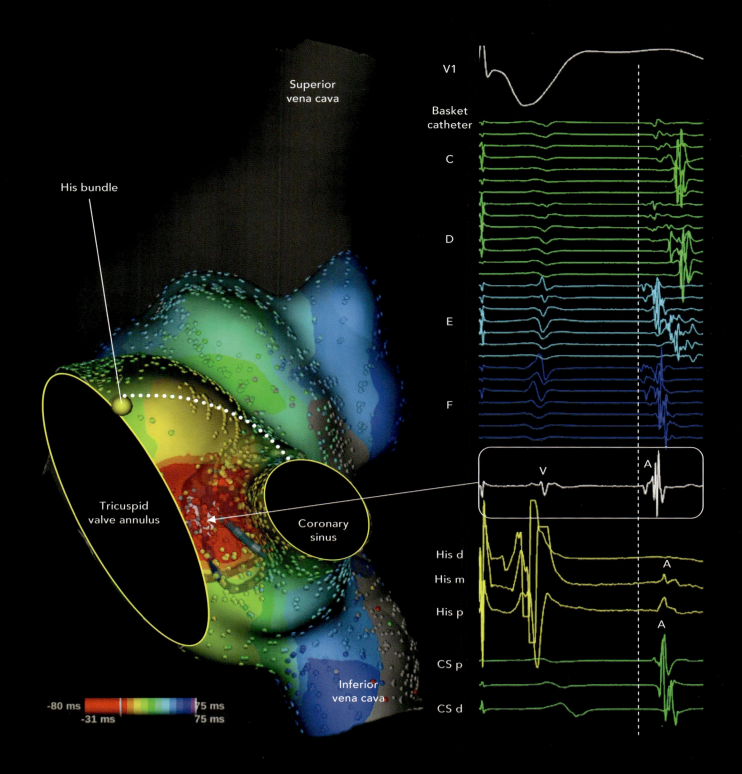

With a jump to slow pathway conduction with long RP, the earliest activation demonstrated by high-resolution mapping is anterior to the coronary sinus orifice. This highlights the anatomic description of the slow pathway as an inferoposterior atrioventricular nodal input. These regions of earliest activation represent the atrionodal connections rather than the actual location of the fast and slow pathways. In both activation maps, the earliest site of activation is diffused, which highlights that these regions may be band-like in nature, rather than discrete fibers.

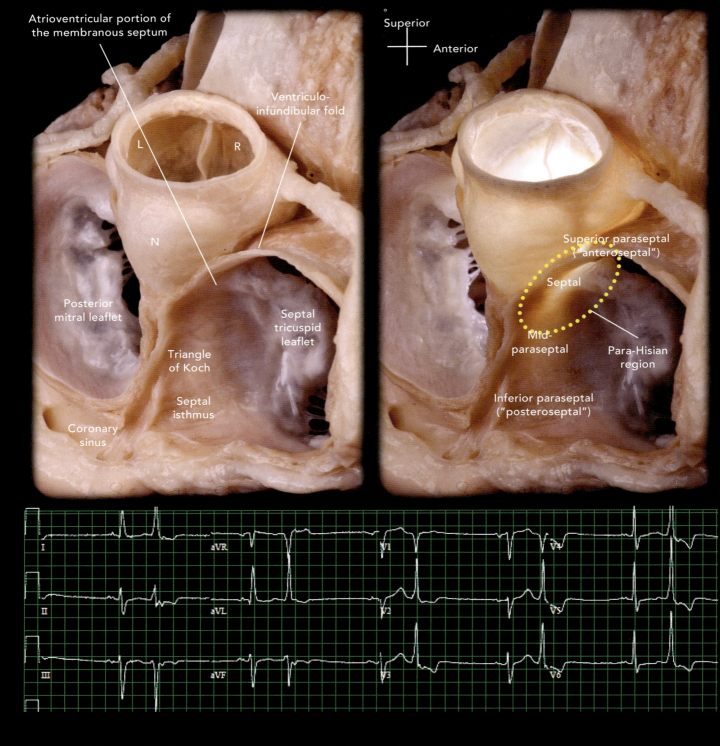

Figures 2-23 and 2-24 *Spotlight*: Para-Hisian region.

Upper panels show attitudinally appropriate terminology to describe the right paraseptal region (right), and their anatomical counterparts (left).[15] Given its close proximity to the conduction system, ventricular arrhythmias originating from the para-Hisian region show relatively narrow QRS. Superior paraseptal origin exhibits an inferior axis. It shows a left or indeterminate bundle branch pattern with early V2 transition with inferior lead discordance with lead II R > III R. Inferior paraseptal origin typically exhibits a superior axis.

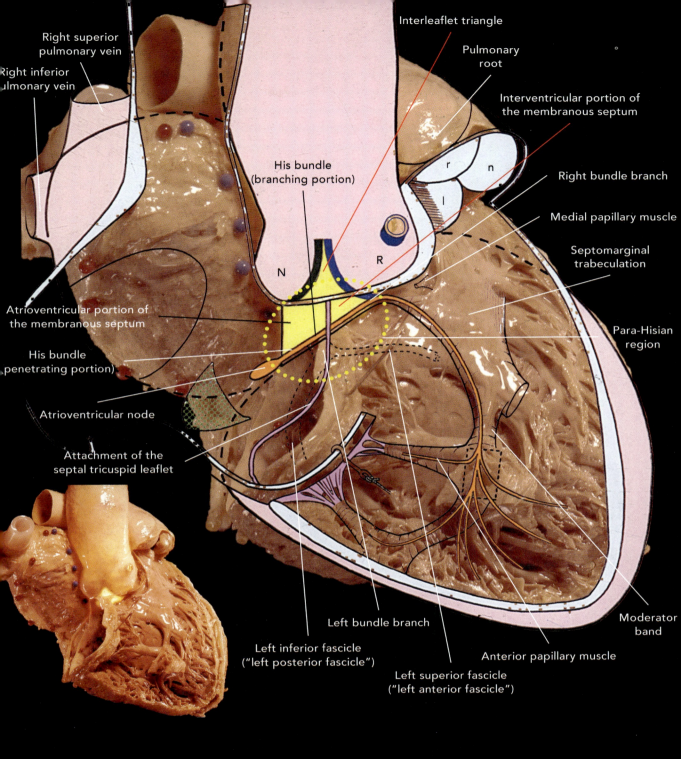

Right superior pulmonary vein

Right inferior pulmonary vein

Interleaflet triangle

Pulmonary root

Interventricular portion of the membranous septum

His bundle (branching portion)

Right bundle branch

Medial papillary muscle

Septomarginal trabeculation

N

R

r

n

l

Atrioventricular portion of the membranous septum

Para-Hisian region

His bundle (penetrating portion)

Atrioventricular node

Attachment of the septal tricuspid leaflet

Moderator band

Left bundle branch

Left inferior fascicle ("left posterior fascicle")

Left superior fascicle ("left anterior fascicle")

Anterior papillary muscle

The para-Hisian region is highly relevant for catheter ablation of atrial tachycardias, accessory pathways, and ventricular arrhythmias. As the His bundle penetrates the central fibrous body before giving rise to the left bundle branch, arrhythmias arising posterior to the His bundle can be considered as atrial and those arising anterior as ventricular. Mapping within the aortic root (noncoronary or right coronary aortic sinuses) is an attractive alternative given the close proximity of the aortic root to the para-Hisian region.

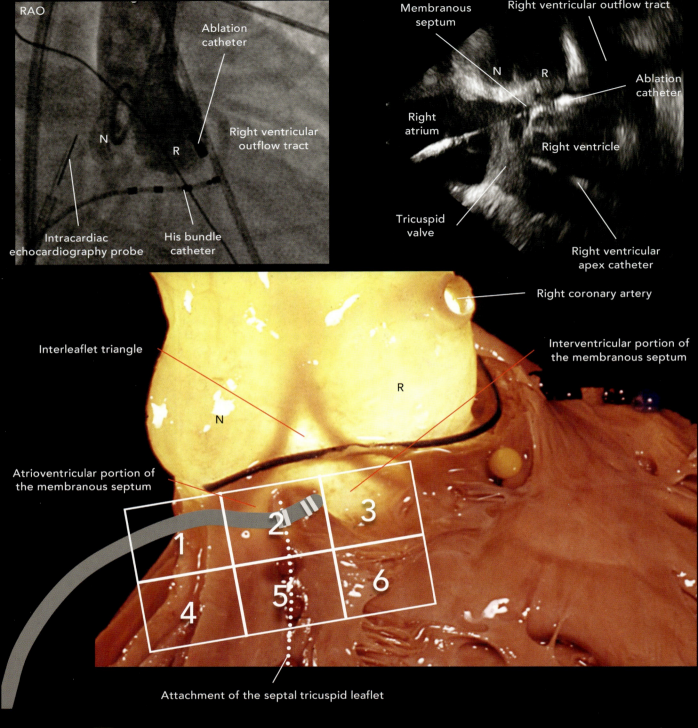

RAO

Ablation catheter

Right ventricular outflow tract

N

R

Intracardiac echocardiography probe

His bundle catheter

Membranous septum

Right ventricular outflow tract

N

R

Ablation catheter

Right atrium

Right ventricle

Tricuspid valve

Right ventricular apex catheter

Right coronary artery

Interleaflet triangle

Interventricular portion of the membranous septum

R

N

Atrioventricular portion of the membranous septum

1

2

3

4

5

6

Attachment of the septal tricuspid leaflet

Figure 2-25 ▶ and Figure 2-26 Six mapping regions around the para-Hisian region.

When mapping arrhythmias in the mid-paraseptal para-Hisian region, this region can be subdivided into six anatomic sections in relation to a near-field His bundle signal (Section 2). The most dangerous section lies inferior and posterior to the His bundle (Section 4), as this indicates the location of the atrioventricular node. In this regard, Sections 5 and 6, which are inferior to the atrioventricular bundle, are the safer regions to ablate. Ablation at Section 3 carries the risk of right bundle branch block (upper right, intracardiac echocardiography).

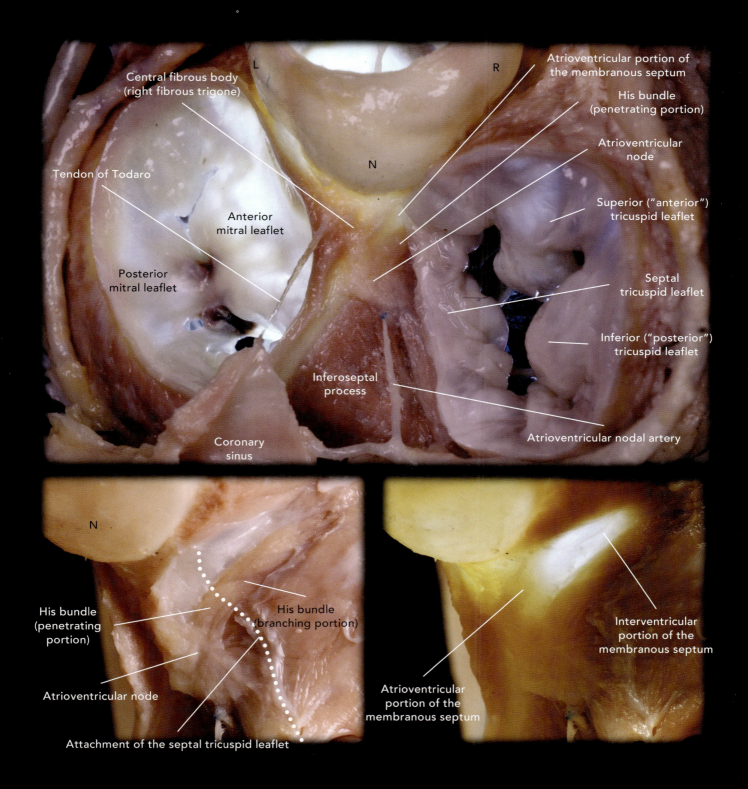

Although ablation at Section 1 is fairly safe, it may injure the atrioventricular node in a case with deep aortic wedging.[16] A noncoronary aortic sinus approach can be an effective and safer alternative. Intracardiac echocardiography is shown with an ablation catheter tip in Section 3 on the home view. The fluoroscopic image with aortic root angiography shows the relationship between the right and noncoronary aortic sinuses and His bundle catheter. Gross dissection images show the three-dimensional feature of the triangle of Koch with the atrioventricular node and His bundle exposed.[17] (See Figures 2-19 and 5-5.)

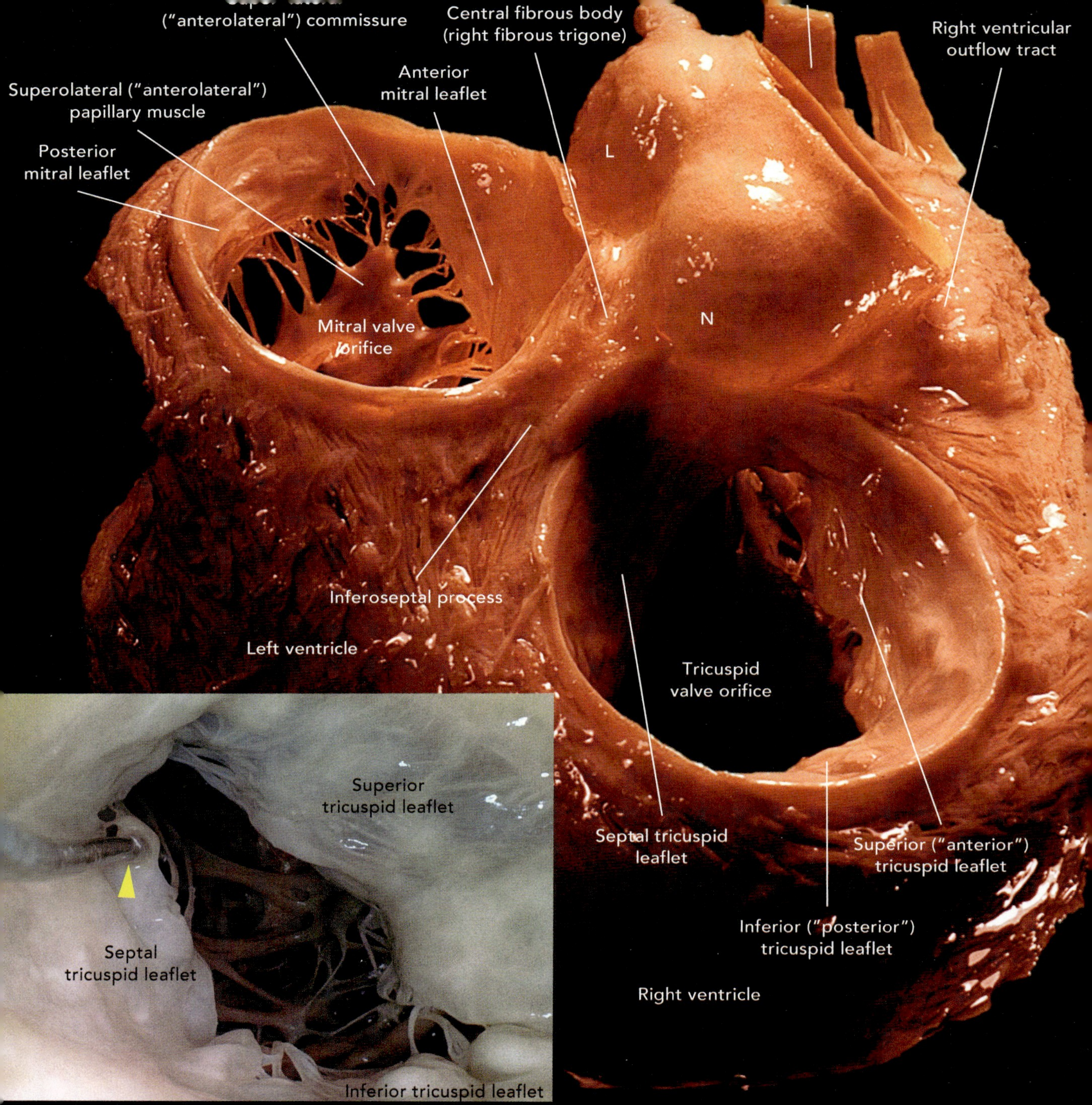

("anterolateral") commissure

Central fibrous body (right fibrous trigone)

Right ventricular outflow tract

Superolateral ("anterolateral") papillary muscle

Anterior mitral leaflet

Posterior mitral leaflet

L

Mitral valve orifice

N

Inferoseptal process

Left ventricle

Tricuspid valve orifice

Superior tricuspid leaflet

Septal tricuspid leaflet

Septal tricuspid leaflet

Superior ("anterior") tricuspid leaflet

Inferior ("posterior") tricuspid leaflet

Right ventricle

Inferior tricuspid leaflet

Figures 2-27 and 2-28   Septal tricuspid leaflet.

The septal tricuspid leaflet can cover the interventricular portion of the membranous septum (Figure 5-9). During permanent pacemaker lead implantation in the His bundle, the septal leaflet may impair fixation insertion, yellow arrowhead). Higher thresholds may be explained by the thin muscular regions with thick fibrous tissues around the membranous septum and motion on the lead imparted by the septal tricuspid leaflet.

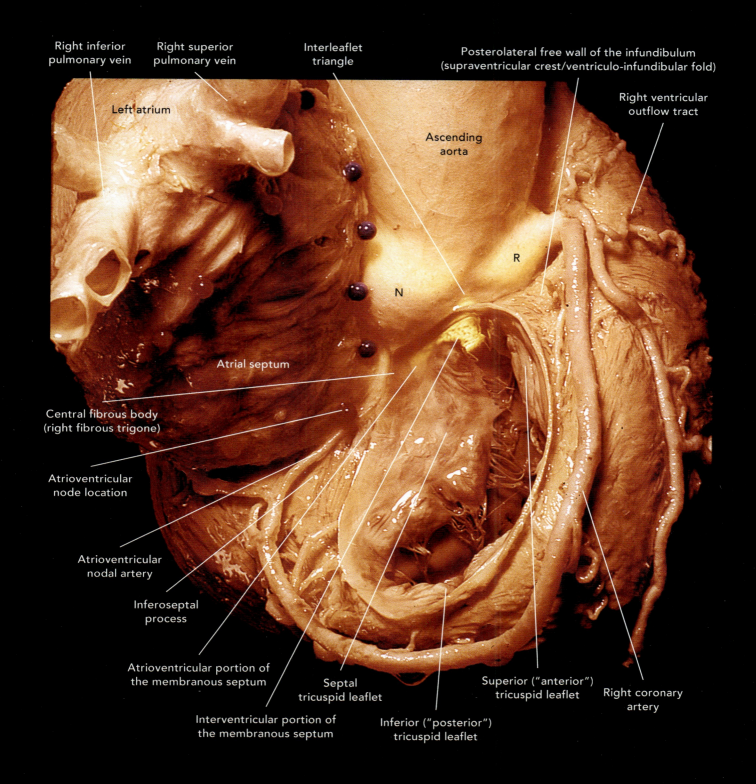

Right inferior pulmonary vein

Right superior pulmonary vein

Interleaflet triangle

Posterolateral free wall of the infundibulum (supraventricular crest/ventriculo-infundibular fold)

Left atrium

Ascending aorta

Right ventricular outflow tract

R

N

Atrial septum

Central fibrous body (right fibrous trigone)

Atrioventricular node location

Atrioventricular nodal artery

Inferoseptal process

Atrioventricular portion of the membranous septum

Septal tricuspid leaflet

Superior ("anterior") tricuspid leaflet

Right coronary artery

Interventricular portion of the membranous septum

Inferior ("posterior") tricuspid leaflet

From the right lateral view after the removal of the right atrium, the atrioventricular nodal artery is seen supplying the atrioventricular node. The penetrating portion of the His bundle within the central fibrous body is located behind the septal attachment of the septal tricuspid leaflet.[18] After penetrating toward the crest of the ventricular septum, the His bundle runs along the inferior margin of the membranous septum located beneath the right and noncoronary aortic sinuses.

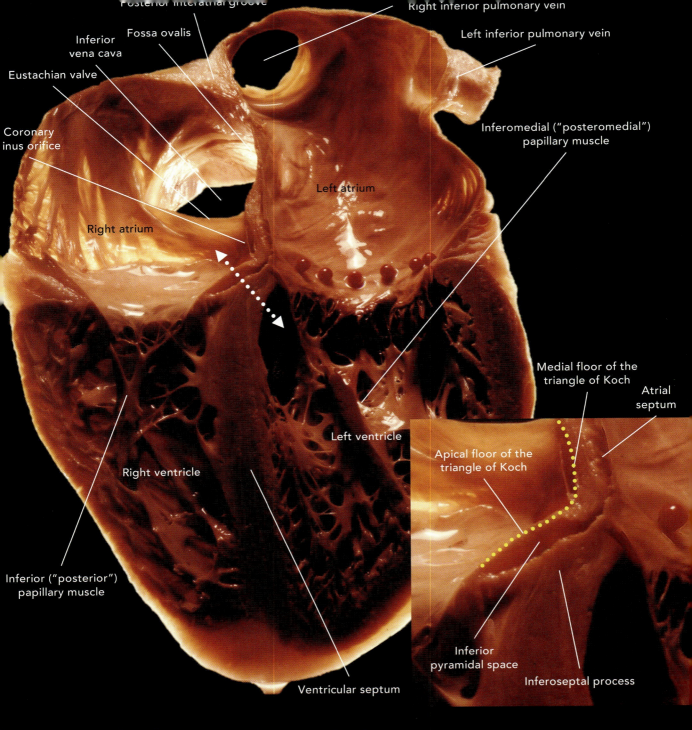

Posterior interatrial groove
Right inferior pulmonary vein
Inferior vena cava
Fossa ovalis
Left inferior pulmonary vein
Eustachian valve
Coronary sinus orifice
Inferomedial ("posteromedial") papillary muscle
Left atrium
Right atrium
Medial floor of the triangle of Koch
Atrial septum
Left ventricle
Apical floor of the triangle of Koch
Right ventricle
Inferior ("posterior") papillary muscle
Inferior pyramidal space
Inferoseptal process
Ventricular septum

Figures 2-29 and 2-30   Atrioventricular sandwich.

The tricuspid valve annulus lies apically to the mitral valve annulus.[7] Because of this offset, the basal inferoseptal left ventricle (inferoseptal process) faces the apical medial right atrium, the apical floor of the triangle of Koch. This region is not the atrioventricular septum, as it is intervened by the epicardial fat of the inferior pyramidal space, including the atrioventricular nodal artery. Thus, this region is referred to as the atrioventricular sandwich. It can be an important vantage point for arrhythmias arising from the inferoseptal process.[19]

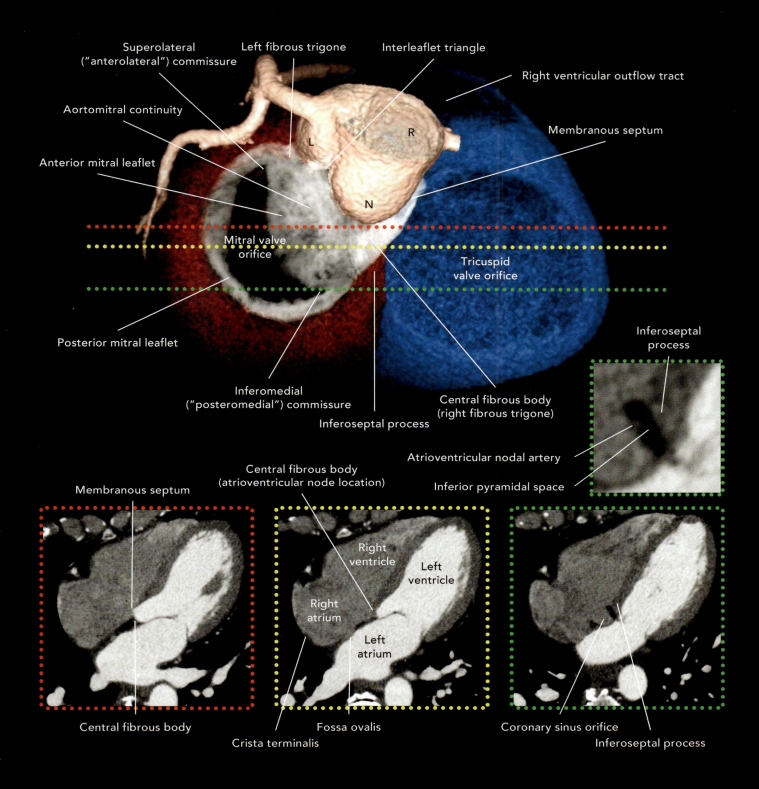

Superolateral ("anterolateral") commissure

Left fibrous trigone

Interleaflet triangle

Right ventricular outflow tract

Aortomitral continuity

Membranous septum

Anterior mitral leaflet

L

R

N

Mitral valve orifice

Tricuspid valve orifice

Inferoseptal process

Posterior mitral leaflet

Inferomedial ("posteromedial") commissure

Inferoseptal process

Central fibrous body (right fibrous trigone)

Atrioventricular nodal artery

Inferior pyramidal space

Membranous septum

Central fibrous body (atrioventricular node location)

Central fibrous body

Crista terminalis

Fossa ovalis

Right ventricle

Left ventricle

Right atrium

Left atrium

Coronary sinus orifice

Inferoseptal process

Further, trans-right atrial access to the left ventricle is feasible via the atrioventricular sandwich in cases with double mechanical valves at the atrioventricular sandwich.[20] Intracardiac echocardiography is useful to guide the procedure. Either congenital[21] or iatrogenic[22] Gerbode-type shunt/fistula/defect should be used as the right atrium-left ventricle communication at the atrioventricular portion of the membranous septum, which is the true anatomical atrioventricular septum. Computed tomographic images show the spatial difference between the atrioventricular septum and the sandwich.

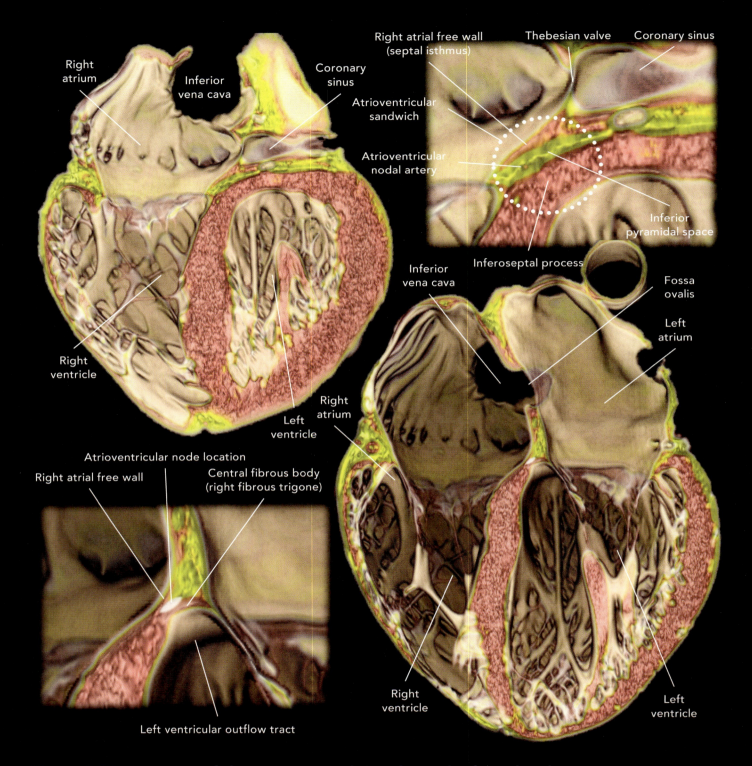

Figure 2-31   Location of the atrioventricular node on the four-chamber view.

A four-chamber view at the level of the coronary sinus orifice shows the atrioventricular sandwich. Note the sandwiched epicardial fat of the inferior pyramidal space, including the atrioventricular nodal artery (upper right inset). A four-chamber view at the level of the central fibrous body just underneath the noncoronary aortic sinus can indicate the potential location of the atrioventricular node (bottom left inset).

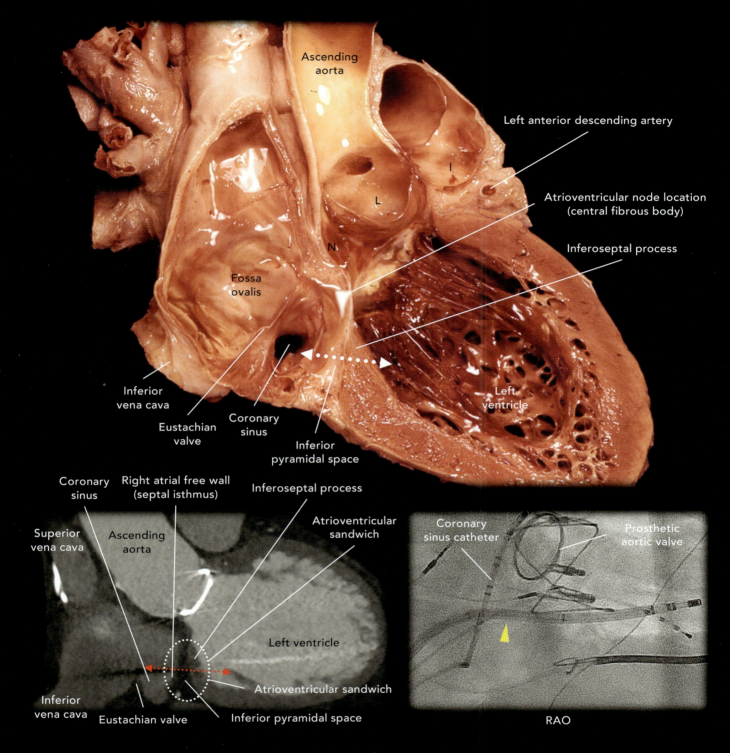

Figure 2-32 **Trans-right atrial access to the left ventricle.**

In a case involving a patient with aortic valve replacement and mitral clip who underwent trans-right atrial access to the left ventricle to ablate the left ventricular arrhythmias, note that the perforation (dotted double-headed arrows, yellow arrowhead) is through the atrioventricular sandwich, involving the apical floor of the triangle of Koch (septal isthmus), inferior pyramidal space, and inferoseptal process.[23] Potential injury to the atrioventricular nodal artery, slow pathway, and risk of cardiac tamponade should be considered as this is the procedure partially exiting the heart. Preprocedural image analysis is fundamental.

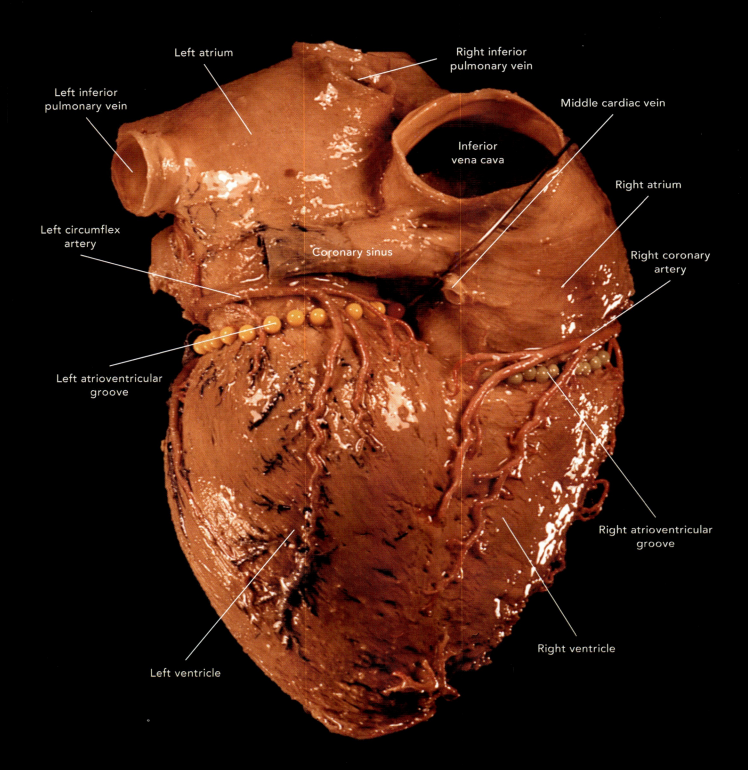

Left atrium

Right inferior
pulmonary vein

Left inferior
pulmonary vein

Middle cardiac vein

Inferior
vena cava

Right atrium

Left circumflex
artery

Coronary sinus

Right coronary
artery

Left atrioventricular
groove

Right atrioventricular
groove

Left ventricle

Right ventricle

Figures 2-33 and 2-34   Inferior crux of the heart.

The crux of the heart is the center, or meeting point, between all four chambers. However, it is not a typical cross due to the offset of the mitral and tricuspid valve annuli. Furthermore, the epicardial fat carrying the atrioventricular nodal artery, referred to as the inferior pyramidal space,[6] wedges deeply toward the central fibrous body. Thus, the epicardial fat is sandwiched between the right atrium and the left ventricle.

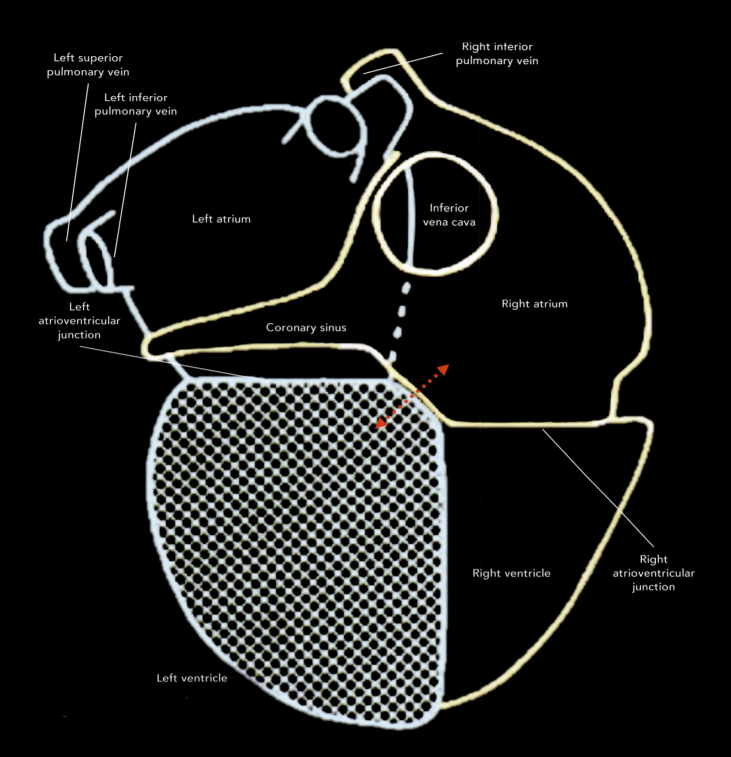

The shared region between the right atrium and left ventricle (red dotted double-headed arrow) is important to understand in the triangle of Koch, inferior pyramidal space, slow pathway modification, ventricular arrhythmias related to the inferoseptal process, and inferior paraseptal accessory pathways.

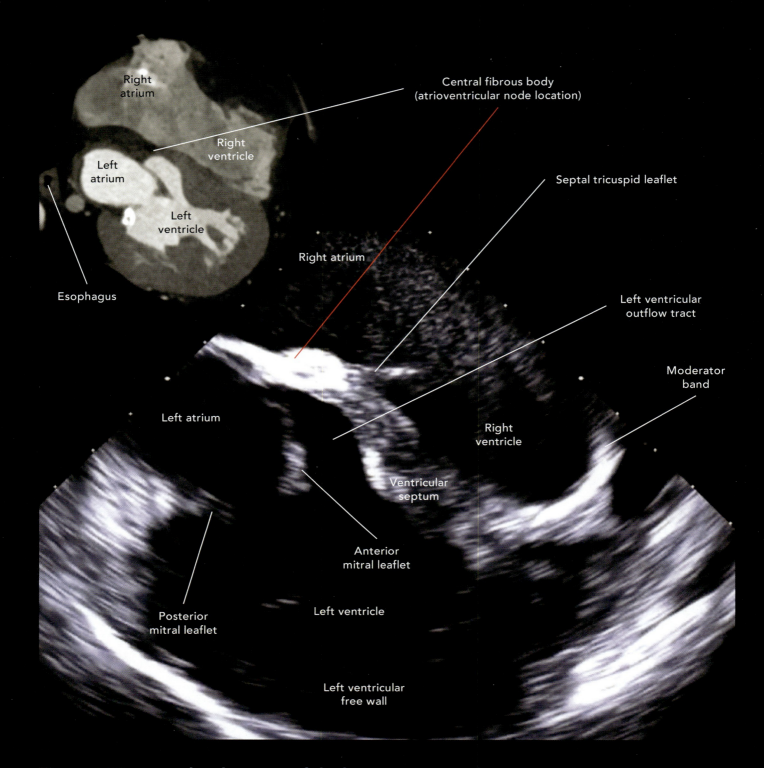

Figure 2-35 **Four-chamber view of the heart on intracardiac echocardiography.**

A four-chamber view at the level of the central fibrous body is achieved by posterior tilt from the basal short-axis view of the aortic valve (Figure 5-18). As this plane involves potential location of the atrioventricular node, basically, the high echogenic area of the central fibrous body is untouchable except for the atrioventricular nodal ablation.

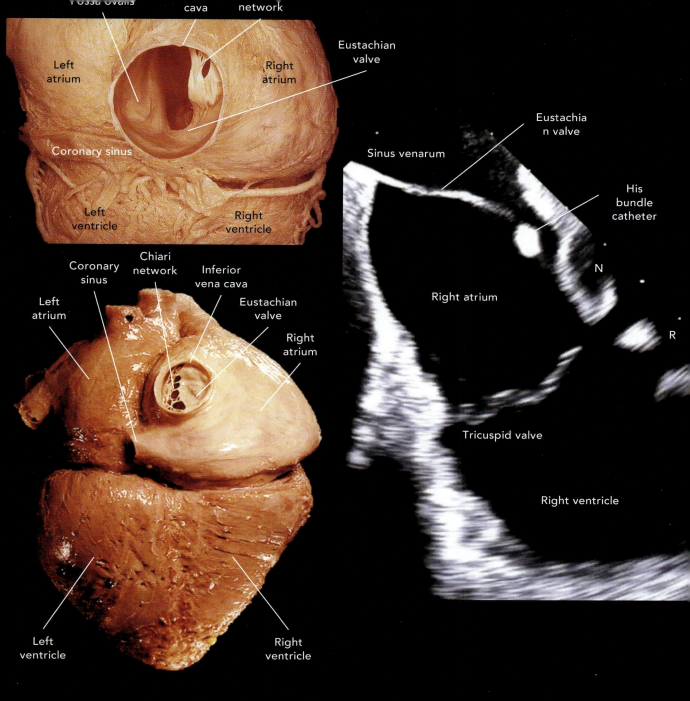

Figure 2-36   Variations of Eustachian valve anatomy.

A prominent Eustachian valve can affect catheter and/or lead manipulation (entrapment, entanglement) into the right atrium and ventricle. A fenestrated Eustachian valve is referred to as a Chiari network. This mobile and redundant structure may often appear like a mobile thrombus and can be traced back on intracardiac echocardiography to the junction of the inferior vena cava and right atrium. The most extreme end of the spectrum for a prominent Eustachian valve is called cor triatriatum dexter because it resembles a distinct third atrium on the right side of the heart.

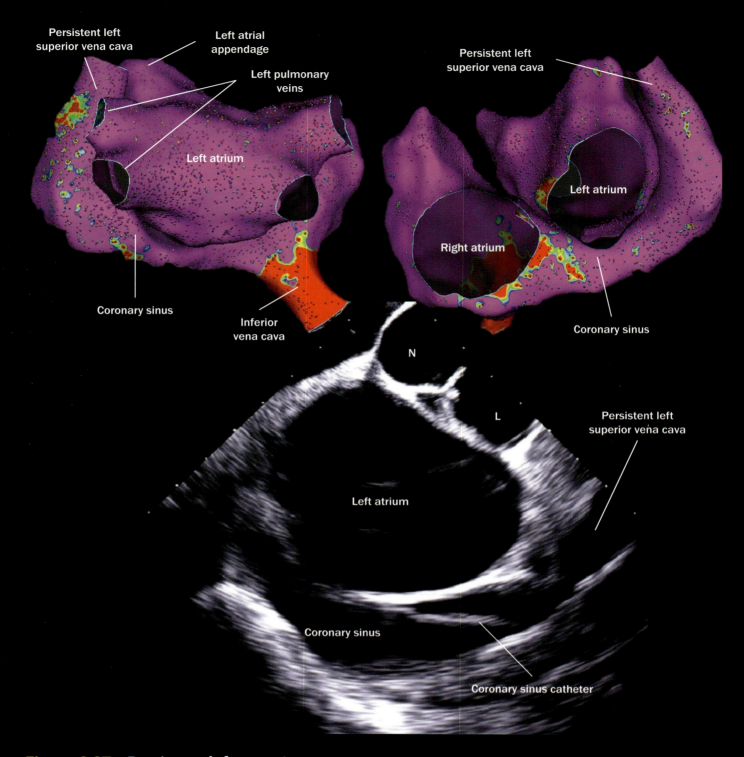

Figure 2-37 **Persistent left superior vena cava.**

Dilation of the coronary sinus can be a diagnostic clue of persistent left superior vena cava. In patients without patent right superior vena cava, device implantation often requires placement of leads into the right ventricle through the persistent left superior vena cava and dilated coronary sinus.[24] In patients with atrial fibrillation, the persistent left superior vena cava may function as a source of triggers that require electrical isolation.[25]

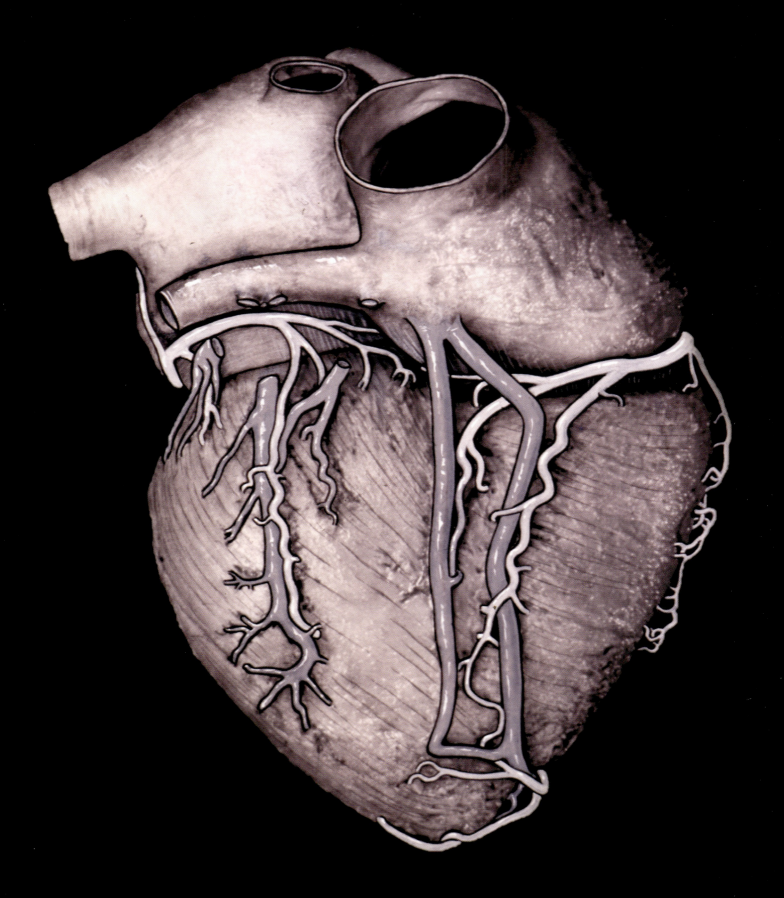

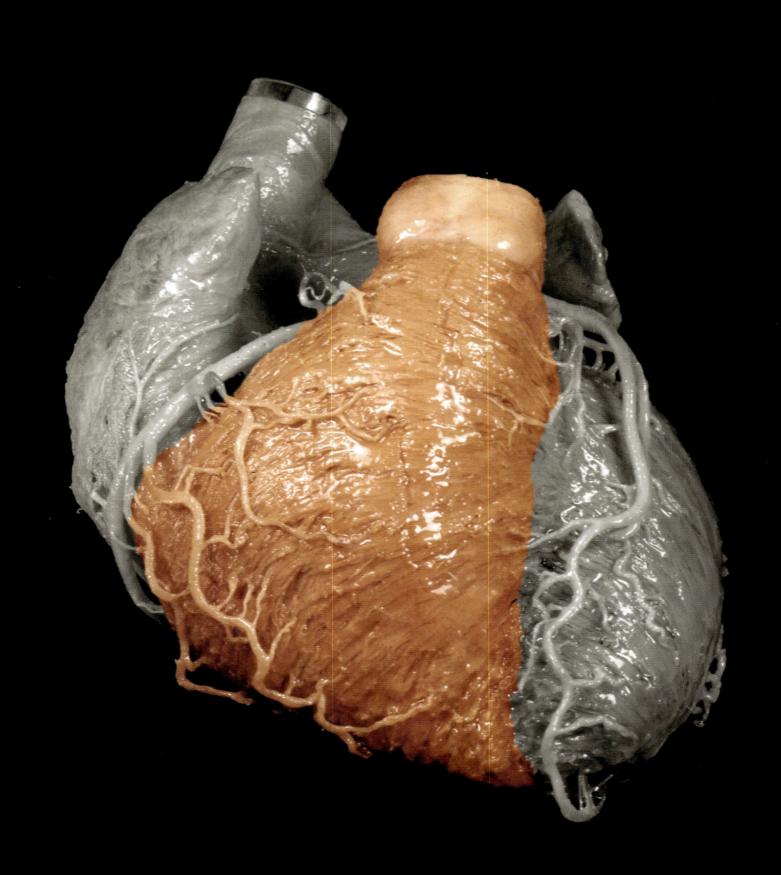

3

The Right Ventricle

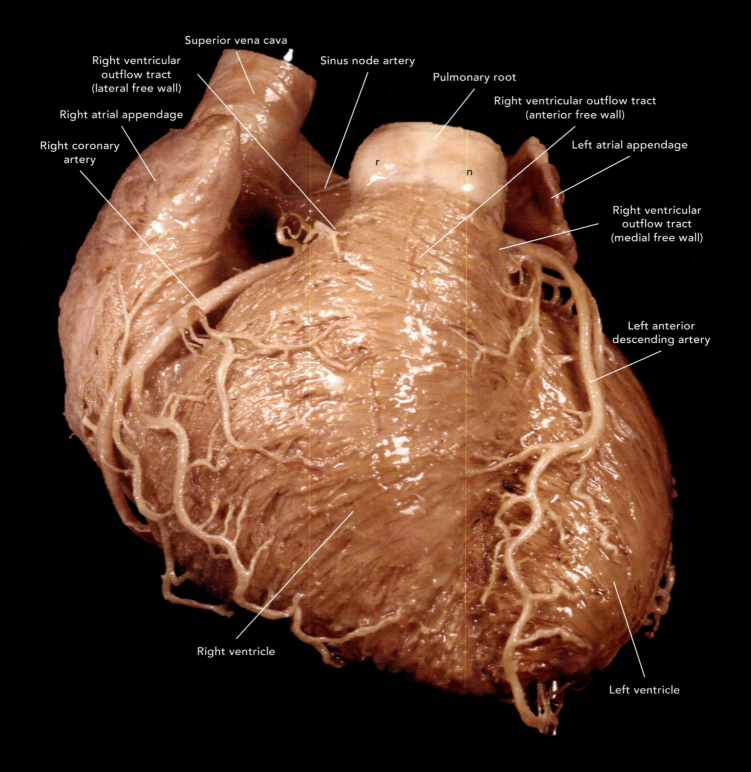

Superior vena cava

Right ventricular outflow tract (lateral free wall)

Right atrial appendage

Right coronary artery

Sinus node artery

Pulmonary root

Right ventricular outflow tract (anterior free wall)

Left atrial appendage

Right ventricular outflow tract (medial free wall)

Left anterior descending artery

Right ventricle

Left ventricle

r

n

Figures 3-1 and 3-2   Frontal view of the right ventricle.

Frontal view of the heart with emphasis on the right ventricle showing an inverted triangular morphology. The anterior free wall of the right ventricle is removed on the right page. This represents the inflow, outflow, and apical trabeculation regions of the right ventricle with the right coronary artery as the lateral boundary and the left anterior descending artery as the septal boundary.

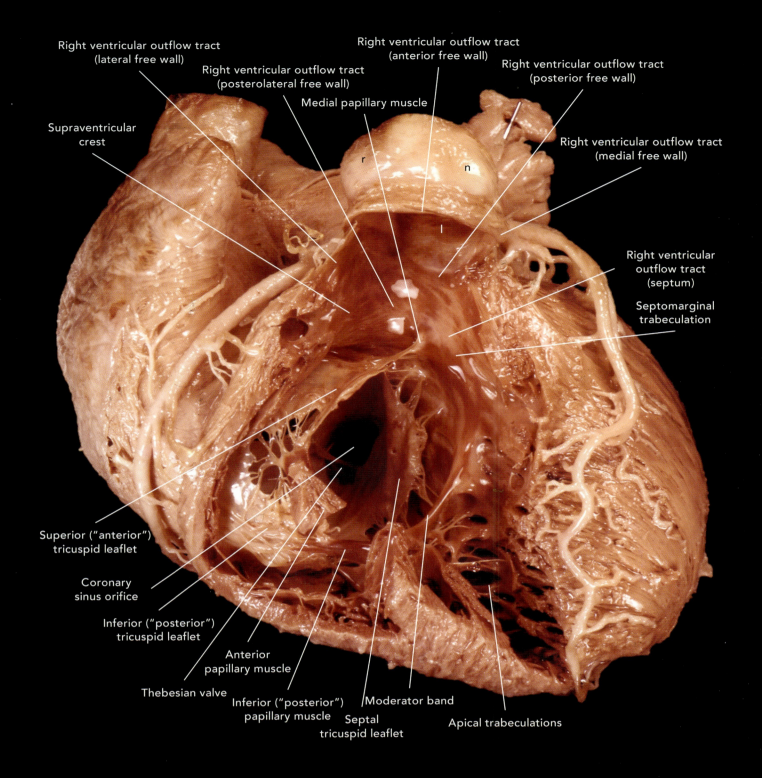

Right ventricular outflow tract (lateral free wall)

Right ventricular outflow tract (posterolateral free wall)

Medial papillary muscle

Right ventricular outflow tract (anterior free wall)

Right ventricular outflow tract (posterior free wall)

Right ventricular outflow tract (medial free wall)

Supraventricular crest

r

n

l

Right ventricular outflow tract (septum)

Septomarginal trabeculation

Superior ("anterior") tricuspid leaflet

Coronary sinus orifice

Inferior ("posterior") tricuspid leaflet

Anterior papillary muscle

Thebesian valve

Inferior ("posterior") papillary muscle

Septal tricuspid leaflet

Moderator band

Apical trabeculations

The moderator band is seen originating from the septomarginal trabeculation, carrying the right bundle branch toward the base of the anterior papillary muscle. The three papillary muscle components are visually within the subvalvular view. The medial papillary muscle lies on the basal septomarginal trabeculation where the supraventricular crest merges with it. The medial papillary muscle gives the chordae tendineae to the medial superior tricuspid leaflet. The largest anterior papillary muscle seen here is sectioned, showing only its head. The inferior papillary muscle lies on the inferior aspect of the right ventricle.

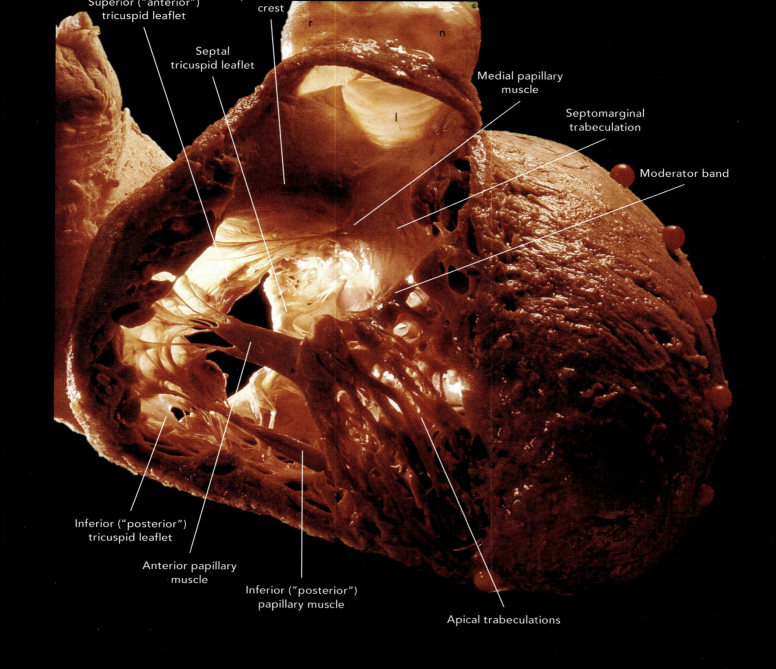

Figures 3-3 and 3-4 labels: Superior ("anterior") tricuspid leaflet, crest, Septal tricuspid leaflet, Medial papillary muscle, Septomarginal trabeculation, Moderator band, Inferior ("posterior") tricuspid leaflet, Anterior papillary muscle, Inferior ("posterior") papillary muscle, Apical trabeculations

Figures 3-3 and 3-4 Right ventricular trabeculations and papillary muscles.

Additional intracavitary view highlighting the moderator band is clearly visualized on the septum with extension toward the anterior papillary muscle, as a complex. Three intact papillary muscles are beautifully observed. The anterior papillary muscle gives the chordae tendineae to the commissure between the superior and inferior tricuspid leaflets. This image also highlights the characteristic apical trabeculations of the right ventricle.

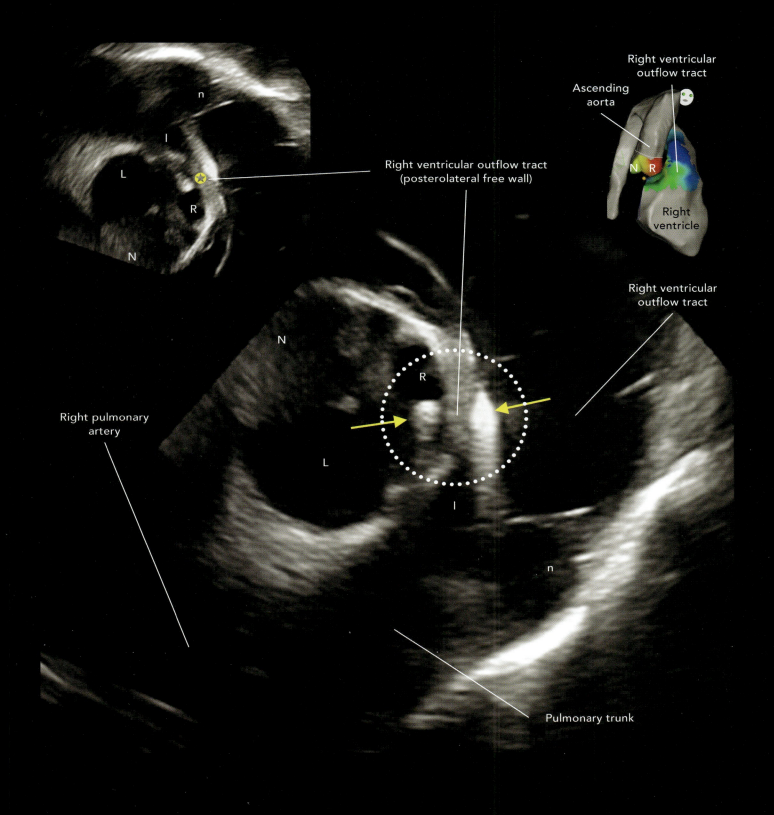

Right ventricular outflow tract (posterolateral free wall)

Right ventricular outflow tract

Ascending aorta

Right ventricular outflow tract

Right ventricle

Right ventricular outflow tract

Right pulmonary artery

Pulmonary trunk

Short-axis view of the aortic valve with intracardiac echocardiography shows convergent catheter profiles. They are placed in the right coronary aortic sinus and right ventricular outflow tract with the posterolateral free wall of the right ventricular outflow tract sandwiched in between. This anatomy suggests the need for careful mapping of the right ventricular outflow tract in a case with ventricular arrhythmia related to the right coronary aortic sinus. The flipped image (upper left) shows an almost identical image with the left-page photograph.

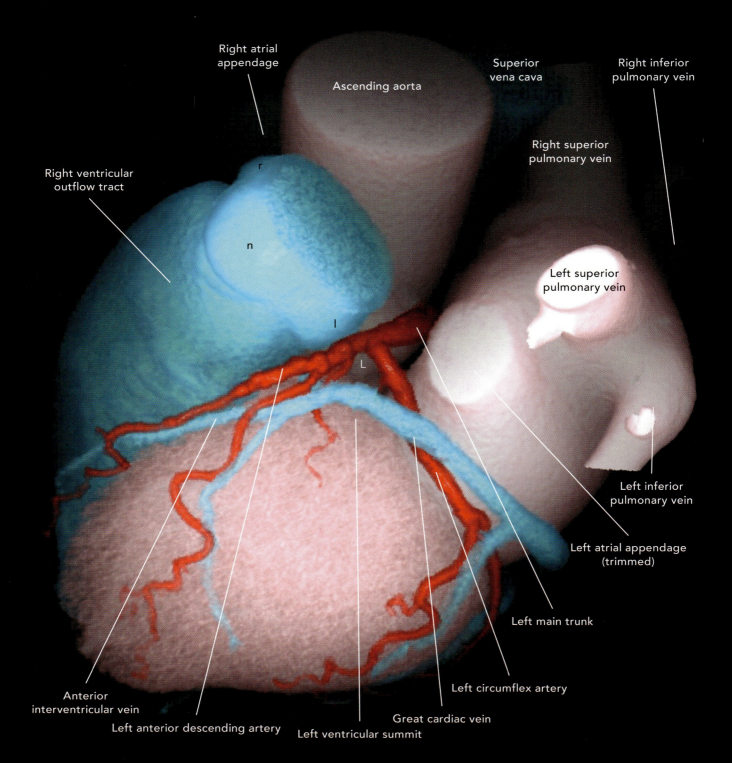

Right atrial appendage

Ascending aorta

Superior vena cava

Right inferior pulmonary vein

Right ventricular outflow tract

Right superior pulmonary vein

r

n

Left superior pulmonary vein

l

L

Left inferior pulmonary vein

Left atrial appendage (trimmed)

Left main trunk

Anterior interventricular vein

Left circumflex artery

Left anterior descending artery

Great cardiac vein

Left ventricular summit

Figures 3-17 and 3-18   **Pulmonary root and the left coronary artery.**

With the pulmonary trunk cut away, the left main trunk becomes apparent just distal to/or at the level of the sinutubular junction of the pulmonary root. It emerges behind the pulmonary root/trunk and immediately anterior to the orifice of the left atrial appendage.

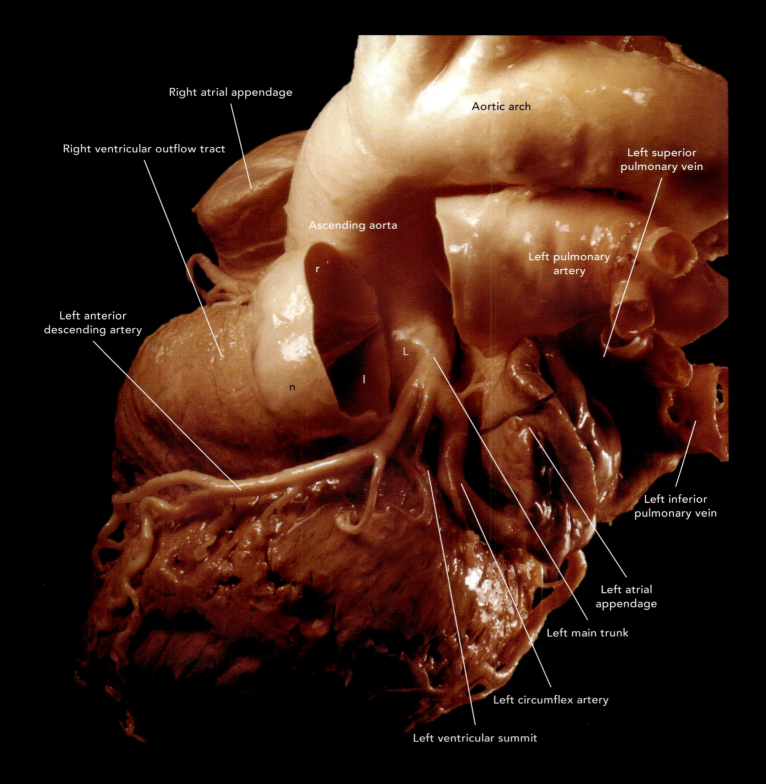

Right atrial appendage

Right ventricular outflow tract

Aortic arch

Left superior
pulmonary vein

Ascending aorta

Left pulmonary
artery

Left anterior
descending artery

r

L

l

n

Left inferior
pulmonary vein

Left atrial
appendage

Left main trunk

Left circumflex artery

Left ventricular summit

The proximal left anterior descending artery skirts the left adjacent pulmonary sinus.[27] Thus, left coronary angiography is strongly recommended before performing ablation within the left adjacent pulmonary sinus.[30] In situ, the proximal left coronary artery is covered and protected by the left atrial appendage (Figure 4-2), which may be a secondary function of the left atrial appendage.

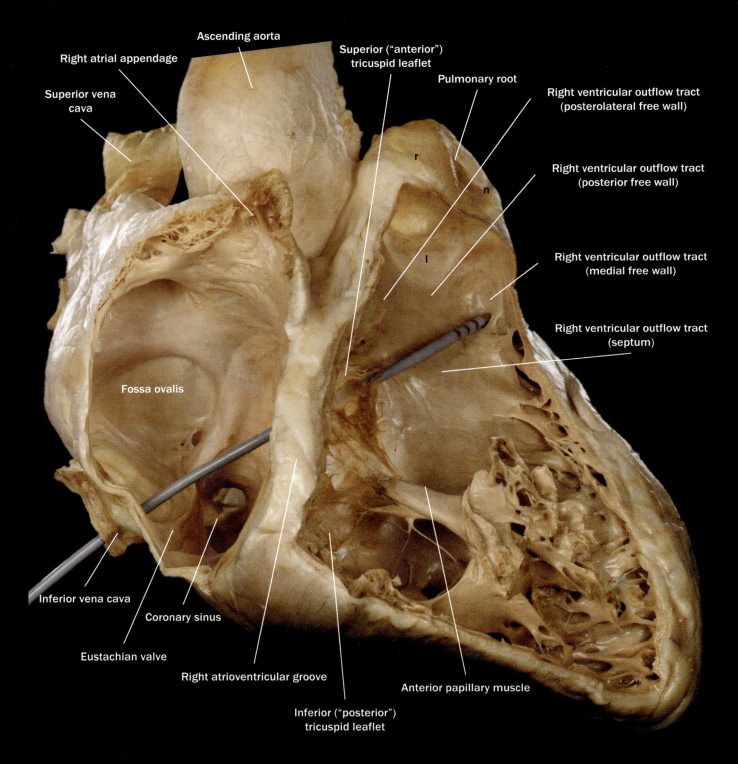

Right atrial appendage

Ascending aorta

Superior ("anterior") tricuspid leaflet

Pulmonary root

Superior vena cava

Right ventricular outflow tract (posterolateral free wall)

Right ventricular outflow tract (posterior free wall)

Right ventricular outflow tract (medial free wall)

Right ventricular outflow tract (septum)

Fossa ovalis

Inferior vena cava

Coronary sinus

Eustachian valve

Right atrioventricular groove

Anterior papillary muscle

Inferior ("posterior") tricuspid leaflet

Figures 3-19 and 3-20   Medial free wall of the right ventricular outflow tract.

In the right (left page) and left (right page) anterior oblique view images, the ablation catheter is placed at the medial free wall of the right ventricular outflow tract. This region, often referred to as the "septal" or "anteroseptal," is not the septum but the thin free wall that abuts the left anterior descending artery.

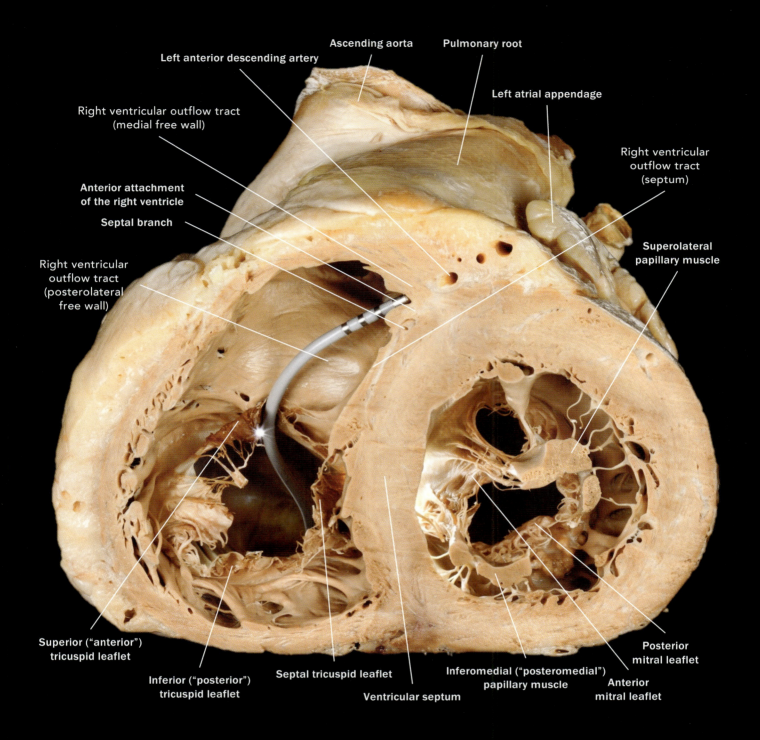

Ascending aorta

Pulmonary root

Left anterior descending artery

Left atrial appendage

Right ventricular outflow tract (medial free wall)

Right ventricular outflow tract (septum)

Anterior attachment of the right ventricle

Septal branch

Superolateral papillary muscle

Right ventricular outflow tract (posterolateral free wall)

Superior ("anterior") tricuspid leaflet

Inferior ("posterior") tricuspid leaflet

Septal tricuspid leaflet

Ventricular septum

Inferomedial ("posteromedial") papillary muscle

Anterior mitral leaflet

Posterior mitral leaflet

This is one of the common sites of right ventricular perforation. Not limited to the outflow tract, this medial free wall near the anterior attachment of the right ventricle (Figure 3-9) is related to perforation and inadvertent injury of the left anterior descending artery.[31]

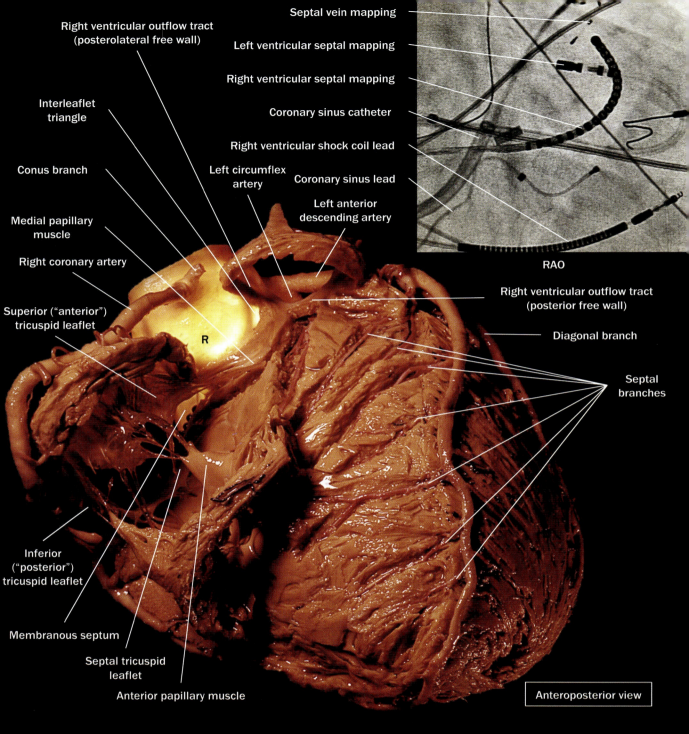

Septal vein mapping

Left ventricular septal mapping

Right ventricular septal mapping

Coronary sinus catheter

Right ventricular shock coil lead

Coronary sinus lead

Left anterior descending artery

Right ventricular outflow tract (posterolateral free wall)

Interleaflet triangle

Conus branch

Left circumflex artery

Medial papillary muscle

Right coronary artery

Superior ("anterior") tricuspid leaflet

R

RAO

Right ventricular outflow tract (posterior free wall)

Diagonal branch

Septal branches

Inferior ("posterior") tricuspid leaflet

Membranous septum

Septal tricuspid leaflet

Anterior papillary muscle

Anteroposterior view

Figures 3-21 and 3-22   Septal perforators.

he basal superior intraseptal region is a challenging region for ablation of ventricular arrhythmias.[32] ypically, patients with mid-myocardial scar may require deeper lesions. The septal perforating veins and rteries provide anatomical vantage points for the intramural portions of the septum.[33] Ethanol injection ay be a method to deliver chemical ablation into the mid-myocardial regions.[34]

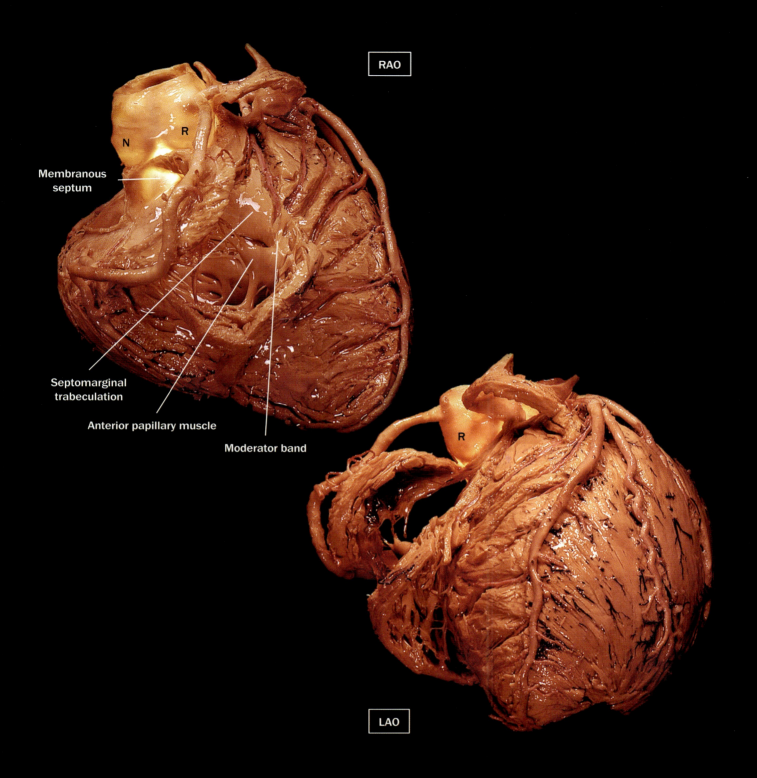

RAO

N R

Membranous
septum

Septomarginal
trabeculation

Anterior papillary muscle

Moderator band

R

LAO

Understanding the dense distribution of these multiple septal branches running deeply inside the ventricular septum also has clinical implications for left bundle branch pacing. Ventricular septal hematoma has been reported as a rare complication of the procedure.[35] Those cases imply that the number of attempts to screw an active fixation lead into the ventricular septum should be minimized as much as possible, or the superior half of the ventricular septum may be better to avoid.

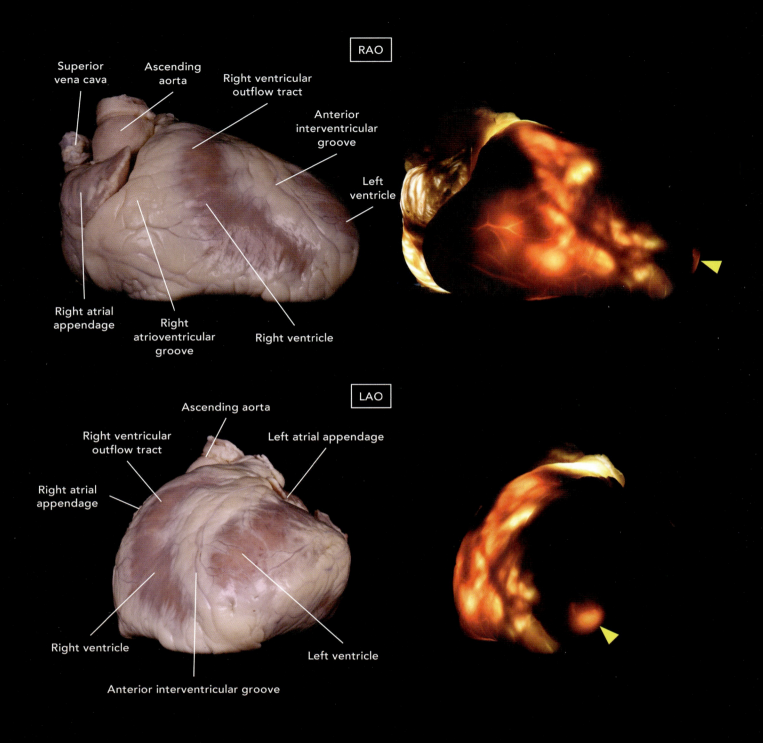

Figure 3-23 **Right ventricular free wall.**

Transillumination revealed the thin free wall of the right ventricle.[4] The apex of the left ventricle is physiologically thin as also revealed by transillumination (yellow arrowheads).[39]

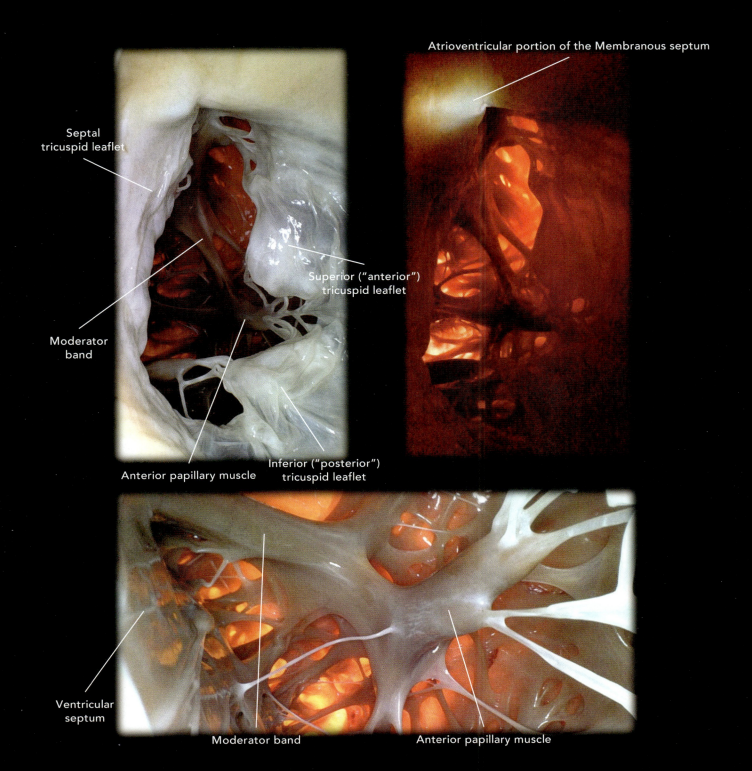

Labels on figure:
- Atrioventricular portion of the Membranous septum
- Septal tricuspid leaflet
- Superior ("anterior") tricuspid leaflet
- Moderator band
- Anterior papillary muscle
- Inferior ("posterior") tricuspid leaflet
- Ventricular septum
- Moderator band
- Anterior papillary muscle

Figure 3-24 **Endoscopic view of the right ventricle.**

The tricuspid valve is viewed from the right atrium (upper left). The light source in the left ventricular outflow tract reveals the location of the atrioventricular portion of the membranous septum (transilluminated in the upper right) at the commissure between the superior and septal tricuspid leaflets. This is where the His bundle catheter is fixed. Further advance into the right ventricle shows the moderator band, anterior papillary muscle, and apical trabeculations. External light source enhances the thin right ventricular free wall.

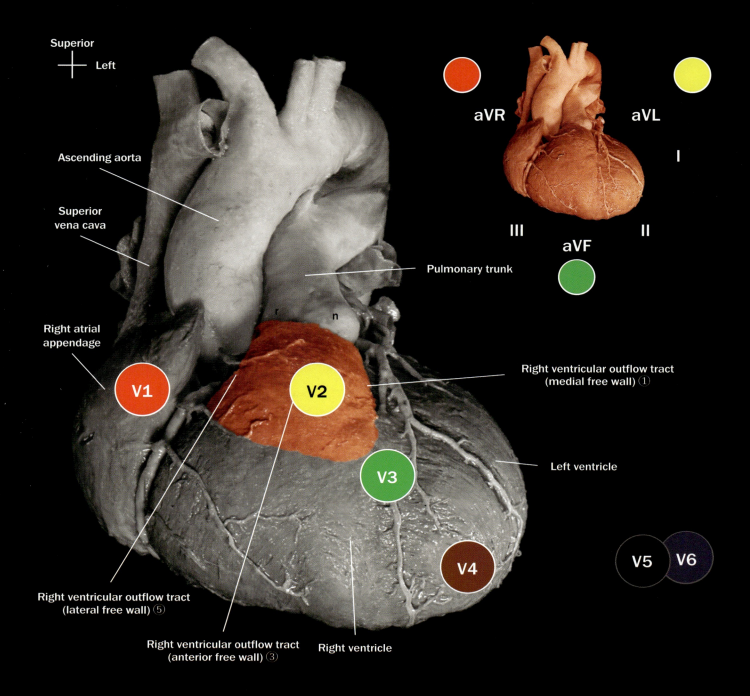

Figures 3-25 and 3-26 **V2 lead location.**

The V2 lead located exactly in front of the right ventricular outflow tract is immediately behind precordial lead V2. V3 lies in the interventricular region, which is why outflow tract arrhythmias with V3 transition may represent right or left outflow tract origins.

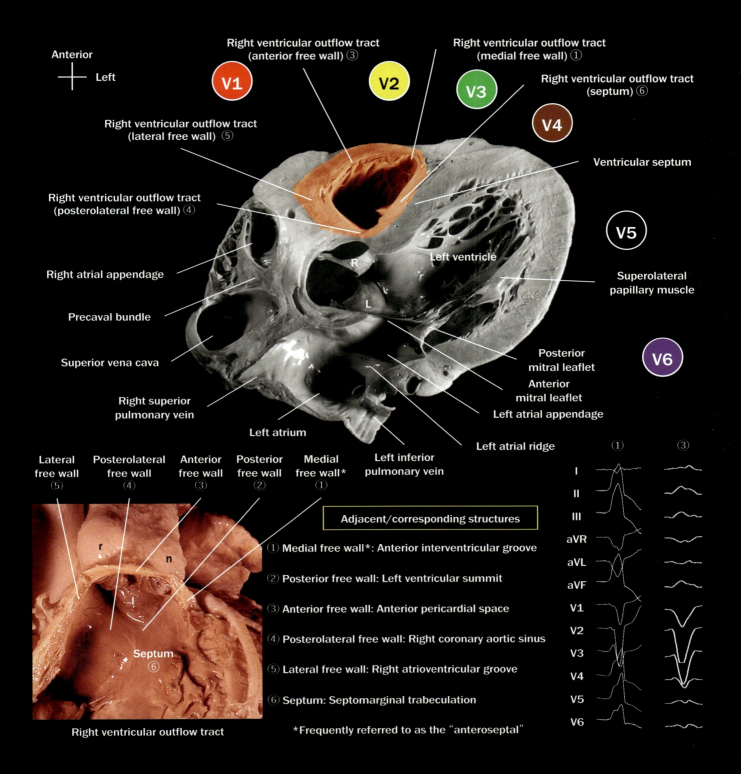

Anterior
┼ Left

Right ventricular outflow tract
(anterior free wall) ③ **V1**

Right ventricular outflow tract
(medial free wall) ①

Right ventricular outflow tract
(medial free wall) ① **V2** **V3**

Right ventricular outflow tract
(septum) ⑥

Right ventricular outflow tract
(lateral free wall) ⑤ **V4**

Ventricular septum

Right ventricular outflow tract
(posterolateral free wall) ④

V5

Right atrial appendage

R

Left ventricle

Superolateral
papillary muscle

Precaval bundle

L

Superior vena cava

Posterior
mitral leaflet

V6

Anterior
mitral leaflet

Right superior
pulmonary vein

Left atrial appendage

Left atrial ridge

Left inferior
pulmonary vein

Left atrium

Posterior
mitral leaflet

Lateral
free wall
⑤

Posterolateral
free wall
④

Anterior
free wall
③

Posterior
free wall
②

Medial
free wall*
①

① ③

I

II

III

aVR

aVL

aVF

V1

V2

V3

V4

V5

V6

Adjacent/corresponding structures

① Medial free wall*: Anterior interventricular groove

② Posterior free wall: Left ventricular summit

③ Anterior free wall: Anterior pericardial space

④ Posterolateral free wall: Right coronary aortic sinus

⑤ Lateral free wall: Right atrioventricular groove

⑥ Septum: Septomarginal trabeculation

*Frequently referred to as the "anteroseptal"

r

n

l

Septum
⑥

Right ventricular outflow tract

The right ventricular outflow tract has six segments. The septal part is located inferoposterior to the right ventricular outflow tract, as the left ventricular outflow tract resides inferoposterior to the right ventricular outflow tract, being overridden in a crisscross fashion. The subpulmonary part is the encircling free wall, which enables the Ross procedure.[40] Understanding the anatomical relationship between each lead position relative to the right ventricular outflow tract is fundamental to understand the QRS morphology of the ventricular arrhythmias originating from each segment.

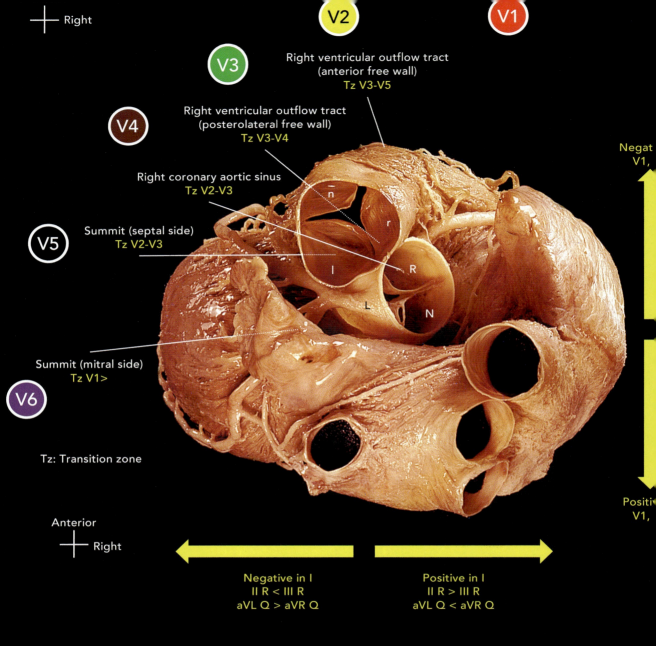

Right

V2

V1

V3

Right ventricular outflow tract
(anterior free wall)
Tz V3-V5

Right ventricular outflow tract
(posterolateral free wall)
Tz V3-V4

V4

Negat
V1,

Right coronary aortic sinus
Tz V2-V3

n

r

Summit (septal side)
Tz V2-V3

V5

I

R

L

N

Summit (mitral side)
Tz V1>

V6

Tz: Transition zone

Positi
V1,

Anterior

Right

Negative in I
II R < III R
aVL Q > aVR Q

Positive in I
II R > III R
aVL Q < aVR Q

Figures 3-27 and 3-28   Electroanatomy of the outflow tracts.

2 lead is located in front of the right ventricular outflow tract, and the left ventricular outflow tr
ocated inferoposterior to the right ventricular outflow tract. Thus, an anterior vector is created fro.
eft ventricular outflow tract, which creates larger R-wave initial amplitudes in V1 and V2. Convers
osterior vector is created from the right ventricular outflow tract, which creates predominantly neg
-waves in V1 and V2.

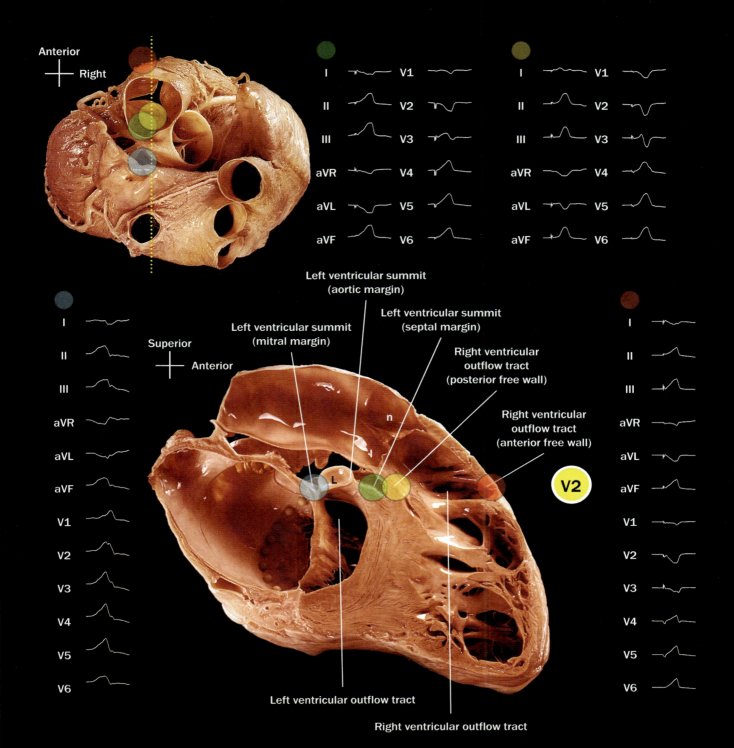

Left ventricular summit (aortic margin)

Left ventricular summit (mitral margin)

Left ventricular summit (septal margin)

Right ventricular outflow tract (posterior free wall)

Right ventricular outflow tract (anterior free wall)

Left ventricular outflow tract

Right ventricular outflow tract

The right lateral view of the sagittal section is useful to understand the structural relationship behind the V2 lead. Note the progressive change observed in the V1–V3 electrodes from the anterior to posterior direction with the transitional zone moving from V3/4 to earlier, while the limb leads show minimal changes. It is surprising how the QRS morphology dramatically changes in such a limited area from the septal margin (green) to the mitral margin (blue) of the ventricular summit.

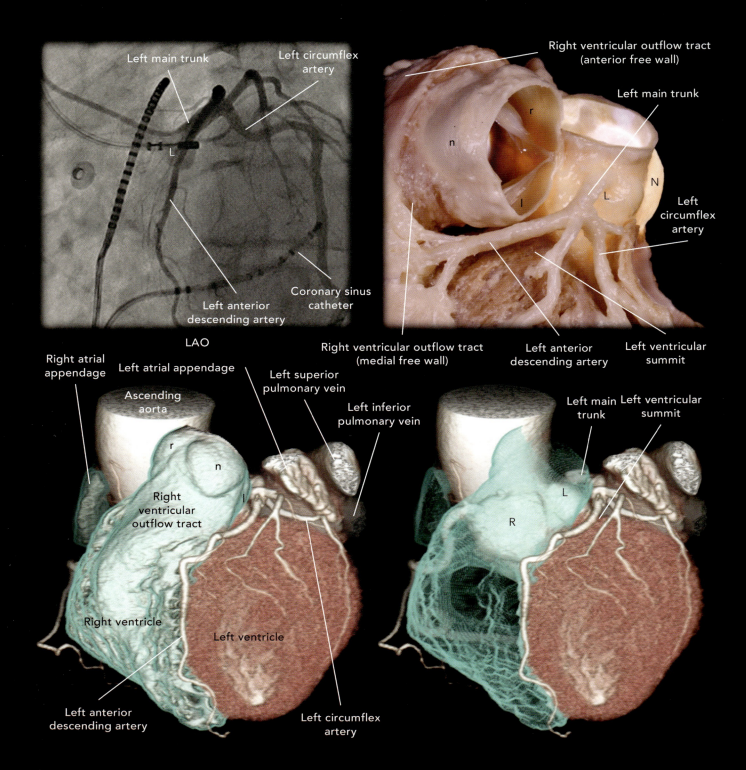

Figure 3-29 **Aortic root and the right ventricular outflow tract.**

A linear mapping catheter and ablation catheter are placed on the anteromedial right ventricular outflow tract and left coronary aortic sinus, respectively (upper left). The right ventricular outflow tract is located leftward and anterior to the aortic root, facing the right coronary aortic sinuses. The interleaflet triangle between the left and right adjacent pulmonary sinuses covers the interleaflet triangle between the right and left coronary aortic sinuses. The adjacent left pulmonary sinus faces the left ventricular summit.

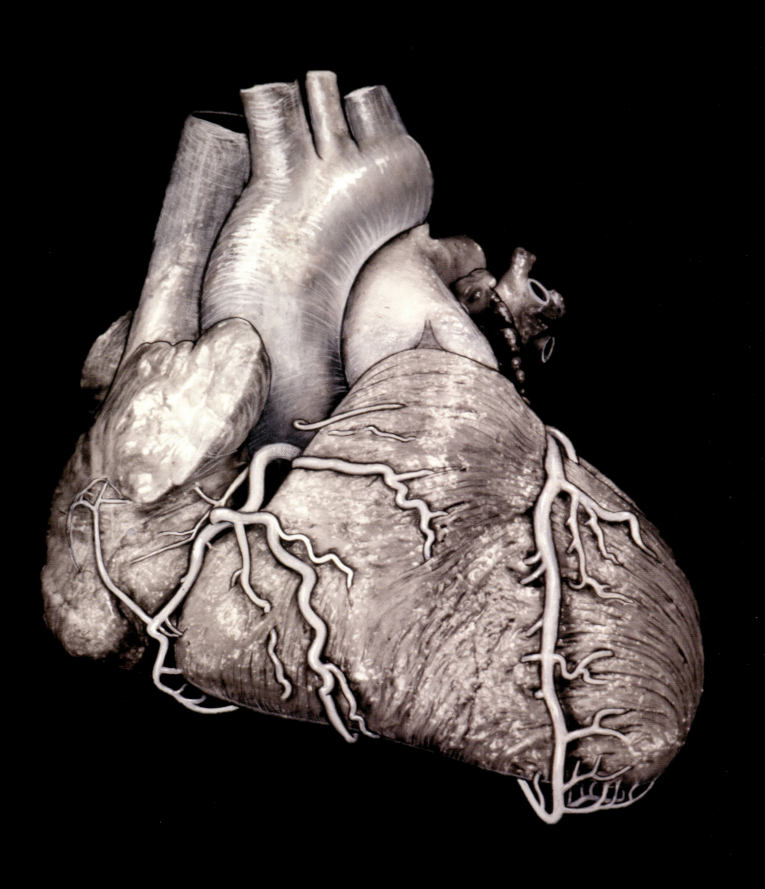

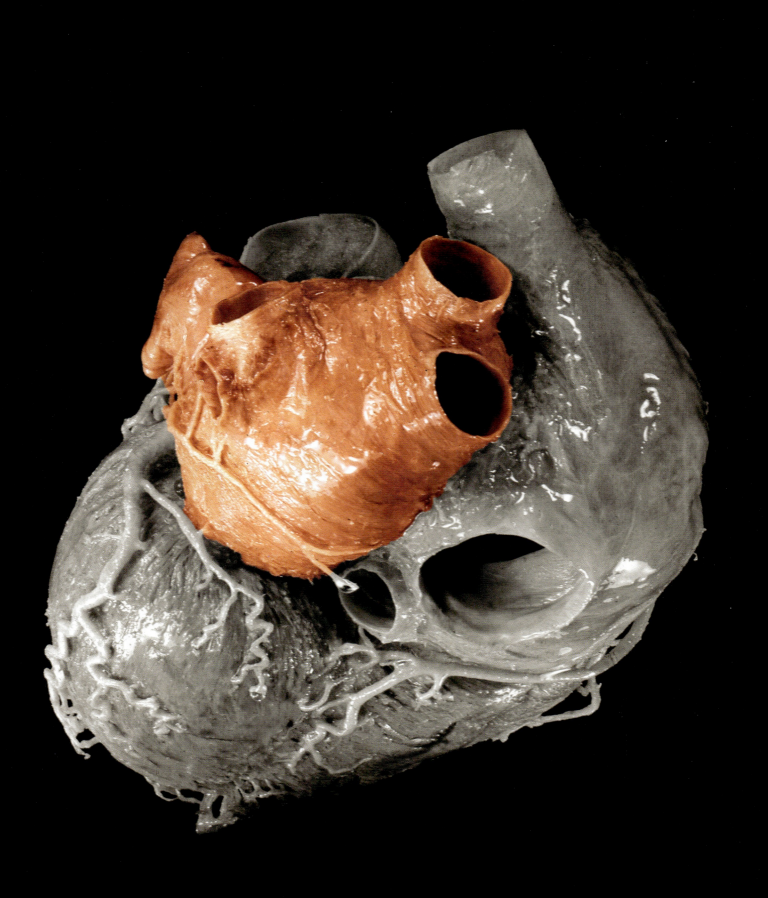

4

The Left Atrium

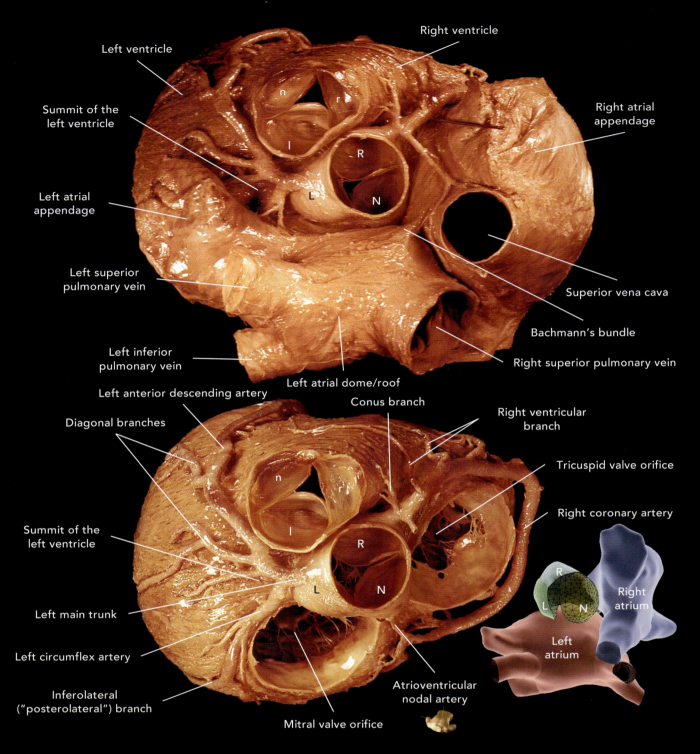

Figure 4-1 **Cranial view of the heart.**

The anterior portion of the right superior pulmonary vein abuts the posteromedial aspect of the superior vena cava. The right phrenic nerve descends close to this region. During pulmonary vein isolation, far-field signals of the superior vena cava can be seen in the right superior pulmonary vein, and differential pacing can be used to confirm isolation. Atrial tachycardias that arise from the right superior pulmonary vein may appear to have the earliest right-sided activation from the medial aspect of the superior vena cava, which requires left-sided mapping to confirm.

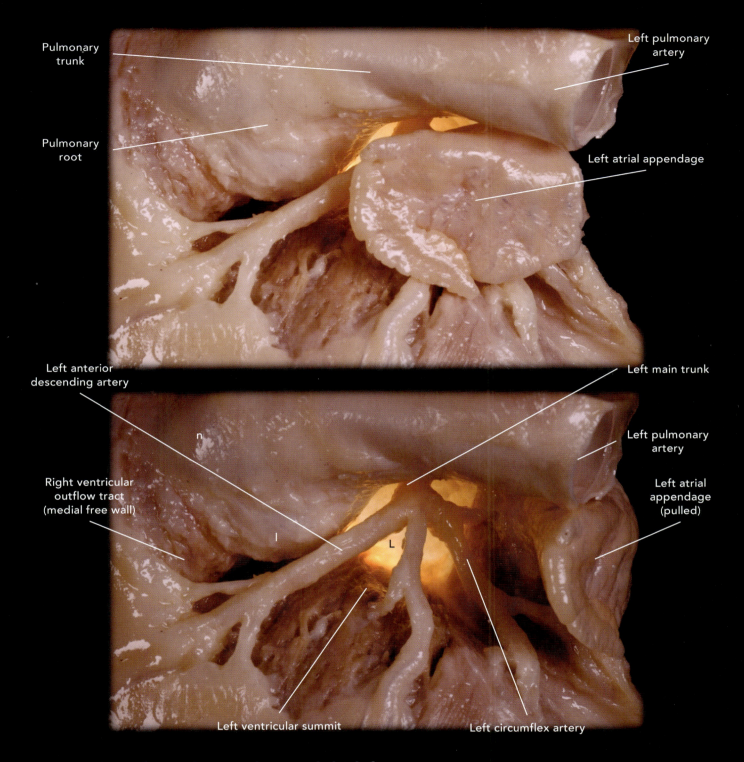

Figure 4-2   Left atrial appendage and the left coronary artery.

The relationship between the left atrial appendage, left ventricular summit, and left coronary artery is highlighted. The compartment surrounded by the left adjacent pulmonary sinus anteriorly, pulmonary trunk superiorly, left atrial anterior wall posteriorly, left atrial appendage laterally, and the left ventricular summit inferiorly is referred to as the left coronary fossa, filled with the epicardial fat surrounding the left coronary artery. Understanding the structural relationship is fundamental for any procedures targeting this three-dimensional area.

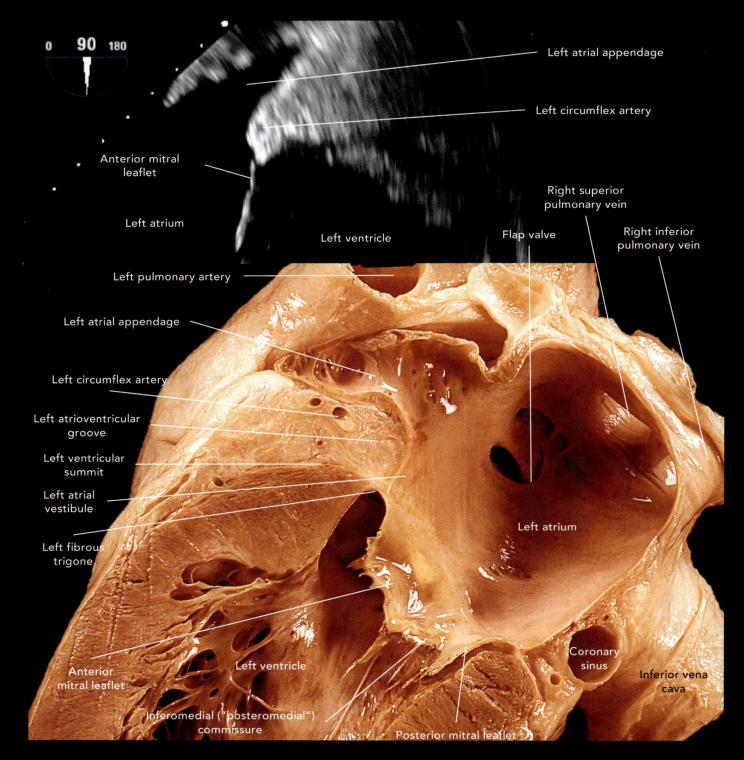

Figure 4-3 **Left atrial appendage regional anatomy.**

The majority of Dr. McAlpine's dissections are photographed after thoroughly removing the epicardial fat. This is one of the rare images where the epicardial fat is preserved within the left coronary fossa. This section, corresponding to the apical two-chamber image, highlights the thickness of epicardial fat between the left atrial appendage and left ventricular summit, which is nearly as thick as the left ventricular wall. This observation implies the limited yield of a percutaneous epicardial approach (Figure 5-26). Corresponding regional anatomy on transesophageal echocardiography is shown (upper).

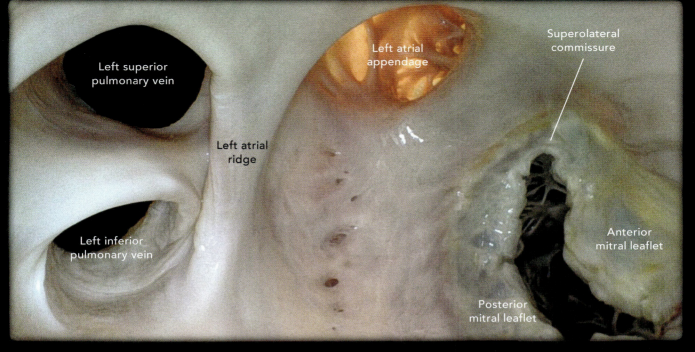

Left superior
pulmonary vein

Left atrial
appendage

Superolateral
commissure

Left atrial
ridge

Left inferior
pulmonary vein

Anterior
mitral leaflet

Posterior
mitral leaflet

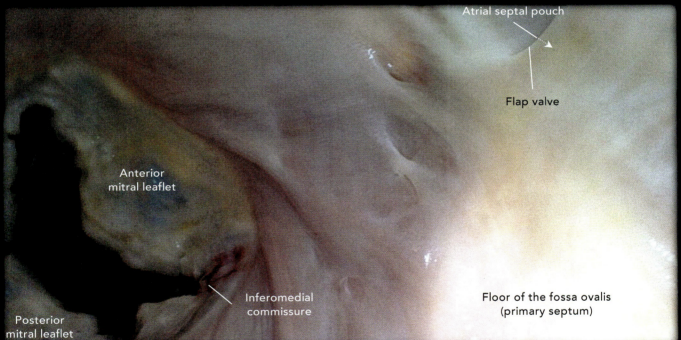

Atrial septal pouch

Flap valve

Anterior
mitral leaflet

Inferomedial
commissure

Floor of the fossa ovalis
(primary septum)

Posterior
mitral leaflet

Figure 4-4 Endoscopic view of the left atrium.

The left atrial appendage orifice is located anterior to the left superior pulmonary vein and resides at 10:00–11:00 of the mitral valve annulus. The left atrial ridge is more prominent at the superior portion than inferior portion. Multiple small diverticula exist below the left atrial appendage orifice, in the mitral isthmus area. The mitral valve opens in an oblique fashion with the superolateral commissure close to the left atrial appendage orifice. The flap valve/atrial septal pouch resides superior to the primary septum (transilluminated), which is related to a patent foramen ovale.

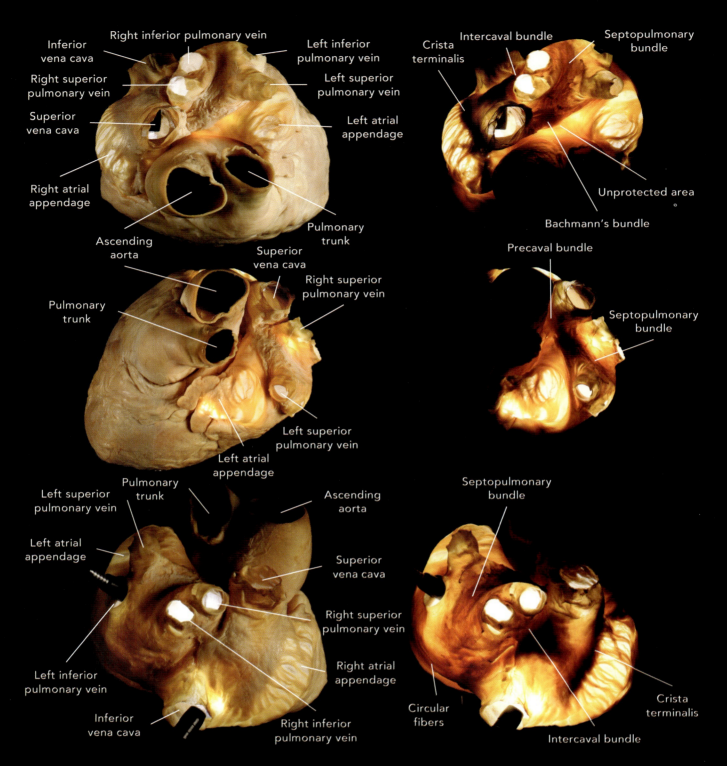

Figure 4-5 **Epicardial fibers and bundles of the left atrium.**

The orientation of the septopulmonary bundle, Bachmann's bundle, intercaval bundle and pectinate muscles within the left atrial appendage, and the fold between the left atrial appendage and the left pulmonary veins (left atrial ridge) are highlighted as the thicker regions compared to the transilluminated area. These structures can render endocardial ablation nontransmural (Figure 4-17).

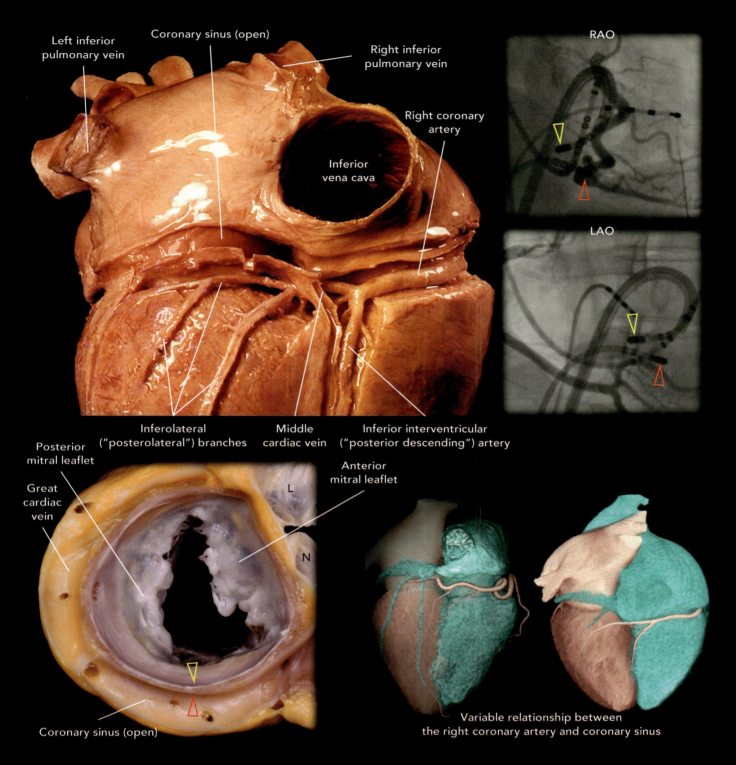

Figure 4-6 *Spotlight:* **Inferior paraseptal accessory pathway.**

The inferior paraseptal ("posteroseptal") region of the left atrium is an important ablation target for accessory pathways. Fluoroscopic images are shown of two approaches: coronary sinus approach (red triangle) and transseptal supravalvular approach with a tight curl (yellow triangle). Ablation of the roof of the coronary sinus carries a higher risk of damage to the fast pathway. When ablation is performed from within the coronary sinus, coronary angiography is necessary to prevent injury to the inferolateral ("posterolateral") branch of the right coronary artery.

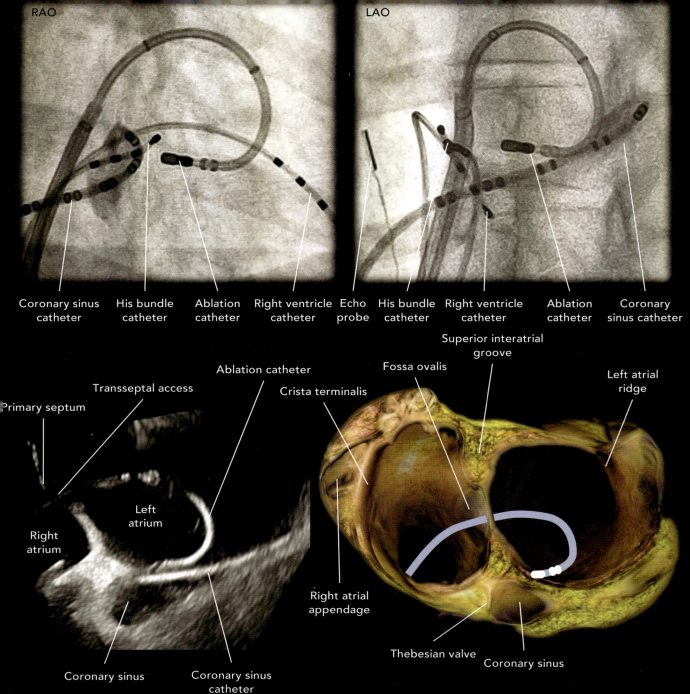

RAO

LAO

Coronary sinus catheter — His bundle catheter — Ablation catheter — Right ventricle catheter — Echo probe — His bundle catheter — Right ventricle catheter — Ablation catheter — Coronary sinus catheter

Primary septum — Transseptal access — Ablation catheter — Crista terminalis — Fossa ovalis — Superior interatrial groove — Left atrial ridge

Left atrium

Right atrium

Right atrial appendage

Coronary sinus — Coronary sinus catheter

Thebesian valve — Coronary sinus

Figures 4-7 and 4-8   Left-sided slow pathway modification.

Aside from inferior paraseptal accessory pathways, ablation of the left-sided slow pathway is conducted from this paraseptal region of the mitral vestibule. Given that the mitral annular plane is basal to the tricuspid plane, larger ventricular electrogram components may be necessary, as the basal left ventricle faces the floor of the triangle of Koch (Figure 2-26). This region is also referred to as the posteromedial left atrial ganglionated plexus region,[11] which is a target of cardioneuroablation for atrioventricular nodal junctional bradycardia.

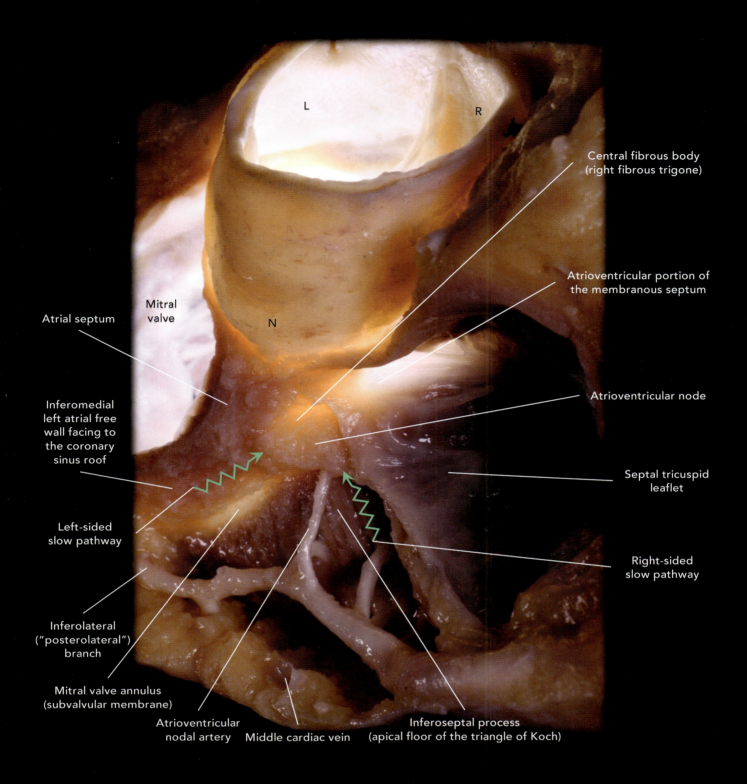

Potential location of the right-sided and left-sided slow pathways, corresponding to the right and left inferior nodal extensions, are illustrated with green arrows. The coronary sinus, located just basal to the right coronary artery, is removed. Note the proximity to the atrioventricular nodal artery ascending behind the floor of the triangle of Koch toward the atrioventricular node. The left slow pathway is likely to be related with the roof of the coronary sinus and the inferomedial free wall of the left atrium facing the inferior pyramidal space.

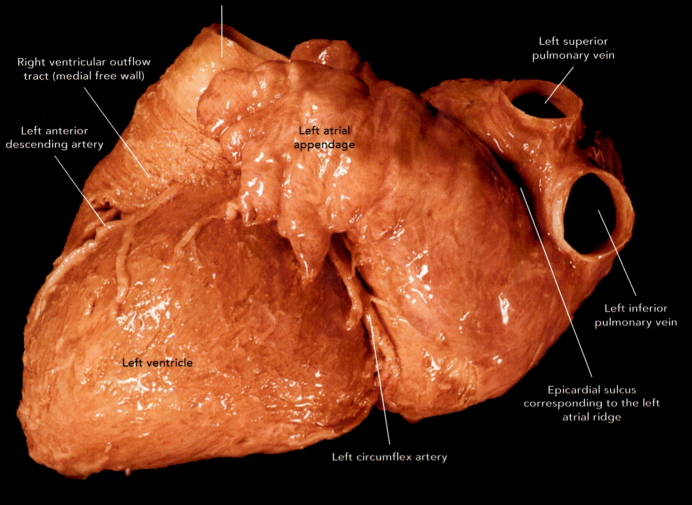

Right ventricular outflow tract (medial free wall)

Left anterior descending artery

Left atrial appendage

Left superior pulmonary vein

Left inferior pulmonary vein

Left ventricle

Epicardial sulcus corresponding to the left atrial ridge

Left circumflex artery

Figures 4-9 and 4-10   Left atrial ridge.

The left atrial ridge, also referred to as the warfarin (Coumadin) ridge, is relevant to pulmonary vein isolation as catheter stability is less optimal. Ablation is often performed on the pulmonary venous side and appendage side of the ridge to achieve transmurality. From an epicardial perspective, this region is a deep fold, with the vein of Marshall (left atrial oblique vein, Figure 4-12) coursing from the coronary sinus in this fold. Left atrial appendage isolation requires extensive ablation along the ridge.

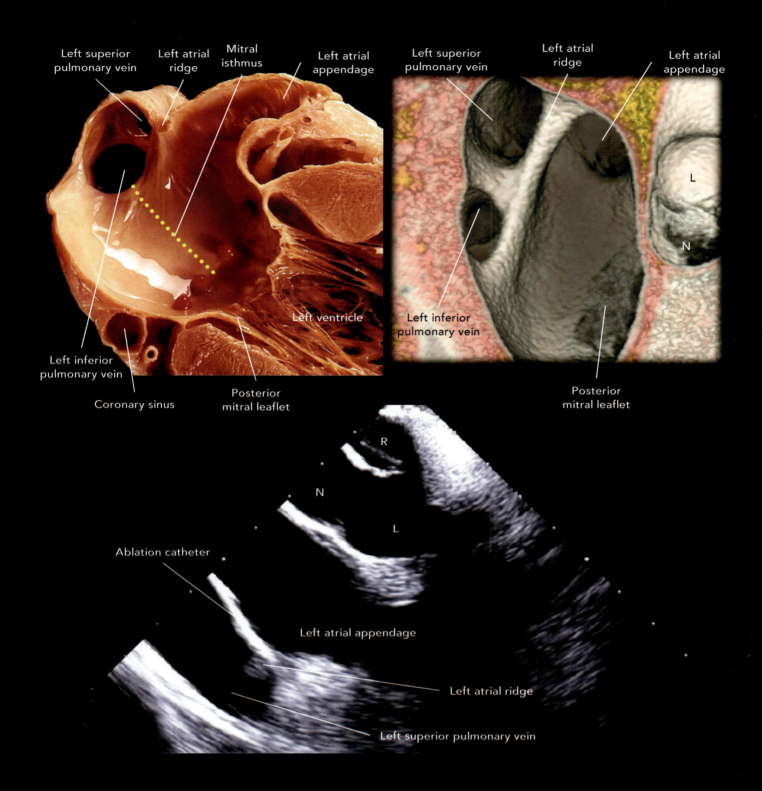

The classical inferior mitral line at the mitral isthmus is shown (dotted yellow line) extending from the left inferior pulmonary vein to the mitral valve annulus. Intracardiac echocardiography visualizes the ridge with the probe placed at the low right ventricular outflow tract, with clockwise rotation from the basal left ventricular view just prior to visualizing the short-axis view of the aortic valve.

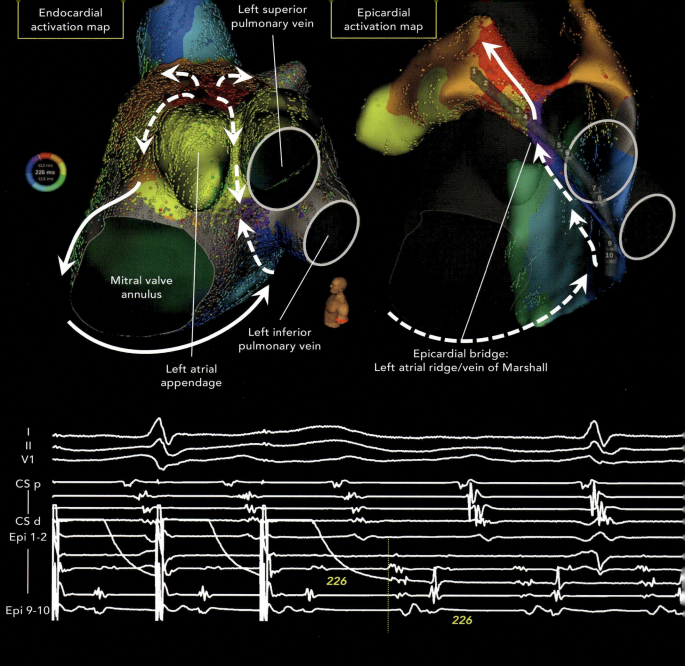

Figures 4-11 and 4-12   **Mitral flutter with epicardial bridging over ridge.**

Case example of an epicardial bridge along the ridge between the left atrial appendage and left pulmona[
veins, involving the vein of Marshall. Endocardial mapping shows a large activation gap in the region c
the prior inferior mitral line. The earliest breakthrough is at the roof after counterclockwise rotation towar
the mitral line (gray). The entire activation gap is recorded within the epicardial fold, corresponding t
the ridge, with a decapolar catheter. Entrainment from the epicardial sulcus overlying the vein of Marsha
confirms participation in the circuit.

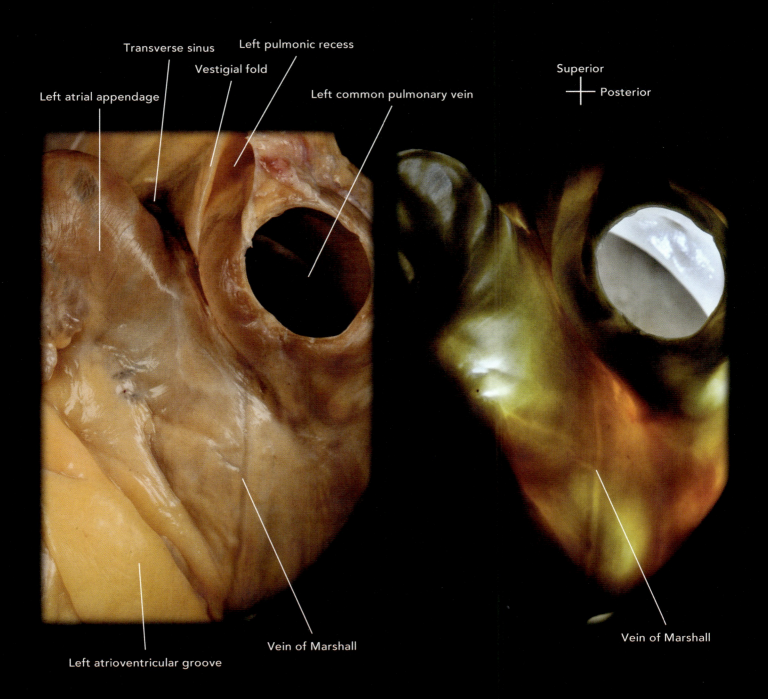

Transverse sinus   Left pulmonic recess

Vestigial fold

Left atrial appendage   Left common pulmonary vein

Superior
Posterior

Vein of Marshall

Left atrioventricular groove

Vein of Marshall

The photographs show a typical and thin vein of Marshall running obliquely on the lateral aspect of the left atrium from the fold between the left atrial appendage and the left pulmonary vein toward the coronary sinus. The superior part is a generally dead-end at the level of the left superior pulmonary vein. The vestigial fold is also referred to as the ligament of Marshall.[41] Multiple epicardial fibers (Marshall bundle) as well as sympathetic nerve fibers have been confirmed along this vein,[42] which can work as the epicardial conduction during pulmonary vein isolation.[43]

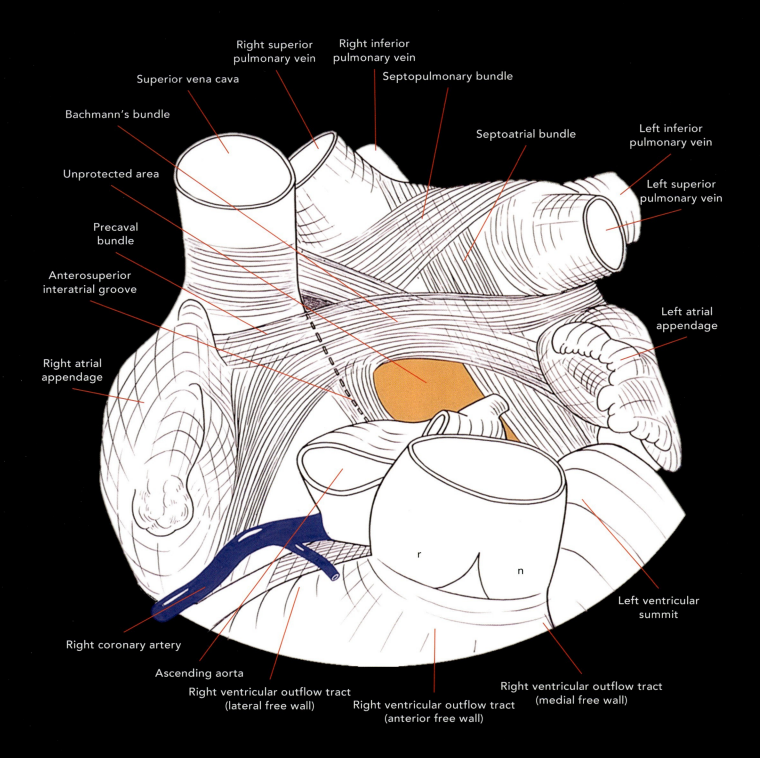

Figures 4-13 and 4-14 **Anterior wall of the left atrium.**

Complex three-dimensional layers of the atrial myofibers are illustrated. The Bachmann's bundle starts from the precaval bundle and runs across the anterosuperior interatrial groove and anterior wall of the left atrium prior to splitting down both sides of the left atrial appendage, into the ridge and toward the mitral valve annulus. The fibers that continue into the ridge is the area of the vein of Marshall. The thinnest region beneath the Bachmann's bundle is immediately posterior to the aortic root, referred to as the unprotected area.

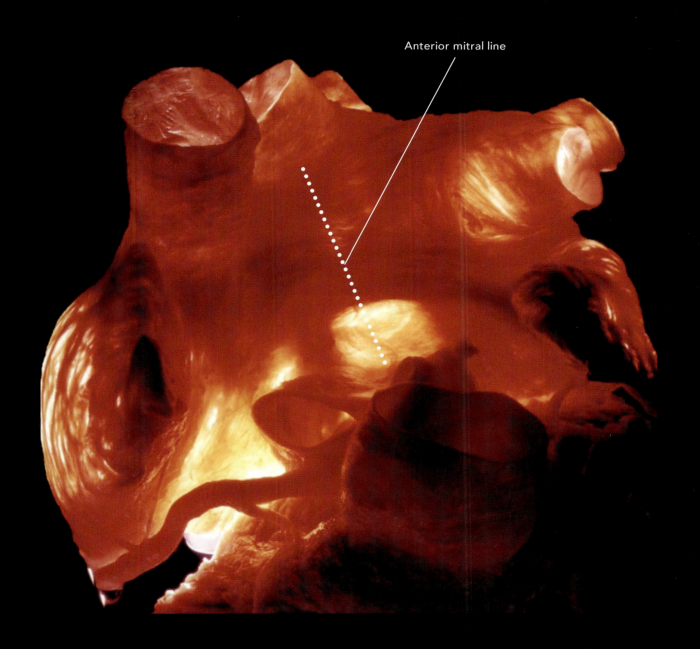

Anterior mitral line

It is likely that nonuniform thickness of the atrial wall (Figure 4-5) contributes to low%–voltage regions using a fixed-amplitude cutoff with contact mapping. Regardless of the location of an anterior mitral line, the Bachmann's bundle region must be transected transmurally, which confounds the ability to block. Note that the thicker portion of Bachmann's bundle is in closer proximity to the interatrial groove and right superior pulmonary vein relative to the mitral valve annulus.

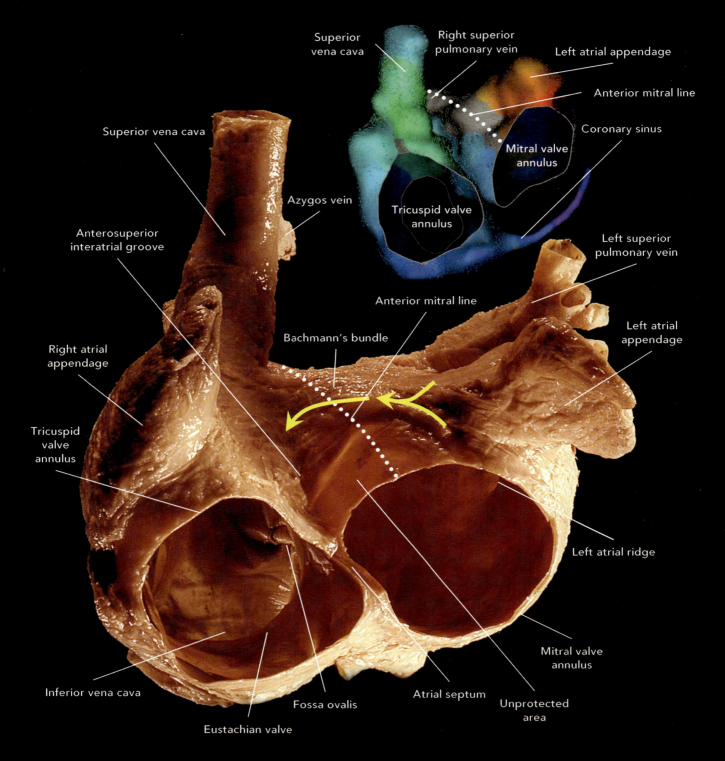

Figure 4-15   Biatrial flutter using the Bachmann's bundle as epicardial bridge.

Incomplete transmurality of an attempted anterior mitral line (white dotted line) results in biatrial flutter during counterclockwise mitral annular flutter. All anterior mitral lines require transmural transection across the Bachmann's region. Bachmann's bundle serves as an epicardial bridge, and the hallmark of this insertion is early focal activation anterior to the superior vena cava in the right atrium. The right atrium, which is typically an outer loop in mitral flutter, becomes an obligatory part of the reentrant loop.

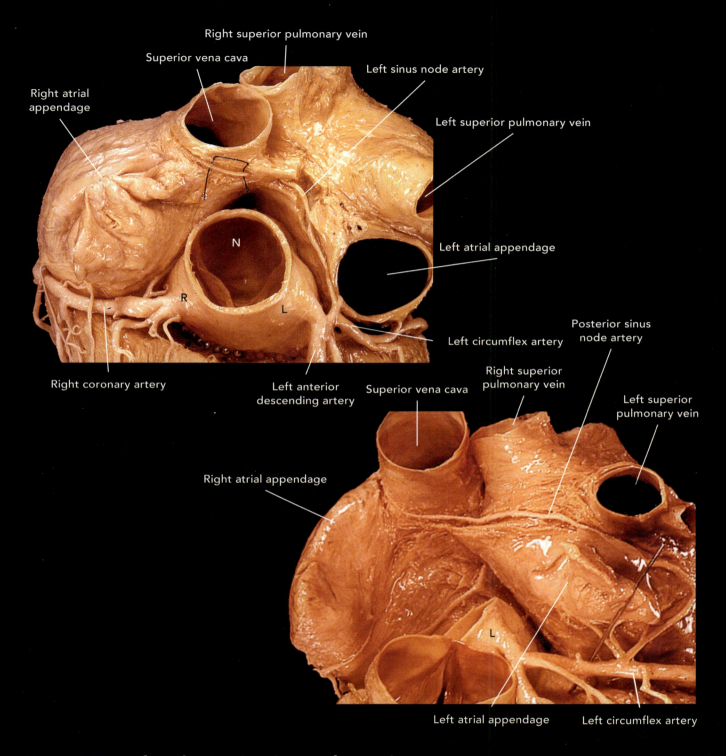

Figure 4-16 **Left and posterior sinus node arteries.**

Although transmural transection across the Bachmann's bundle is required to complete anterior mitral line, approximately 40%–50% of the cases may have sinus node arteries originating from the left circumflex artery.[44] They run directly on the Bachmann's bundle, after coursing either anterior or posterior to the left atrial appendage orifice. Thus, preprocedural evaluation of these arteries is mandatory before attempting transmural transection of the Bachmann's bundle. Note the posterior sinus node artery runs within a fold corresponding to the left atrial ridge.

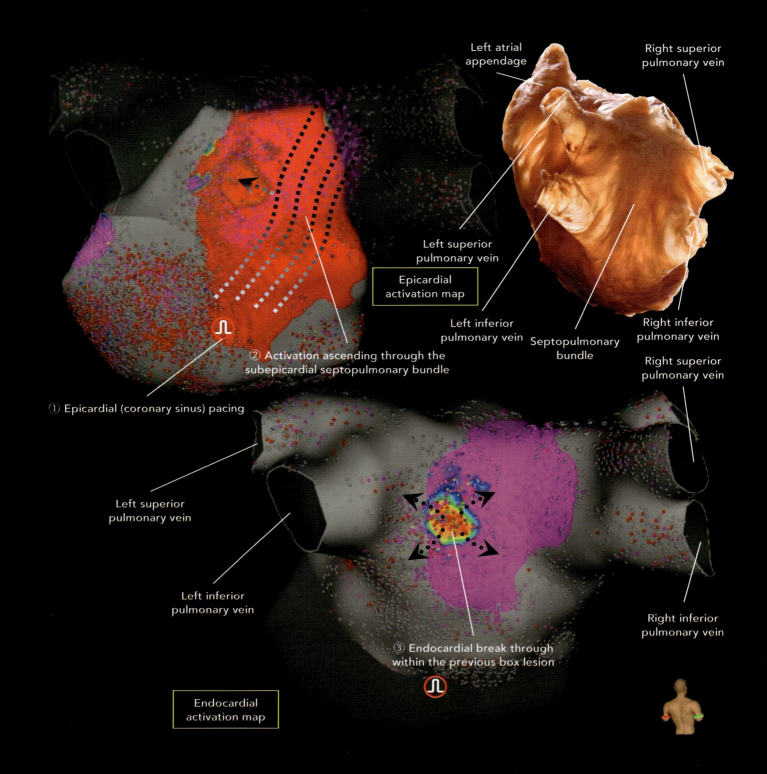

Figure 4-17   Epicardial bridging via the septopulmonary bundle.

The septopulmonary bundle consists of epicardial fibers that originate from the septum and drape over the left atrial dome toward the vestibule. These epicardial fibers impair the ability to isolate the posterior wall with a box lesion set. The hallmark of epicardial bridging via the septopulmonary bundle fibers is focal activation within the center of a box lesion set. Direct epicardial mapping[45] confirms epicardial activation through the septopulmonary bundle and endocardial breakthrough within the previous box lesion set.[46]

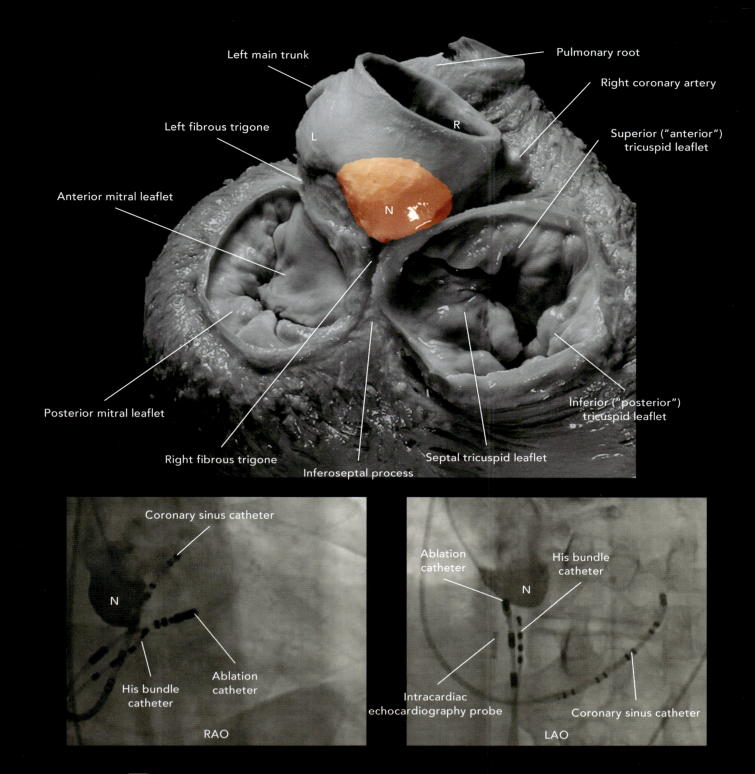

Figure 4-18 ▶ **Noncoronary aortic sinus.**

The noncoronary aortic sinus is clinically considered an atrial structure as it shares a relationship with both the right and left atrial anterior medial free wall (exception, Figure 3-8). Thus, it represents an anatomic vantage point for the anteroseptal aspects of the right and left atria, including the para-Hisian region above the membranous septum (superior paraseptal, Figure 2-23). Fluoroscopic images (bottom) captured during aortic angiography exclusively show the noncoronary aortic sinus in relation to the His bundle catheter. The ablation catheter is placed on Section 3 (Figure 2-25).

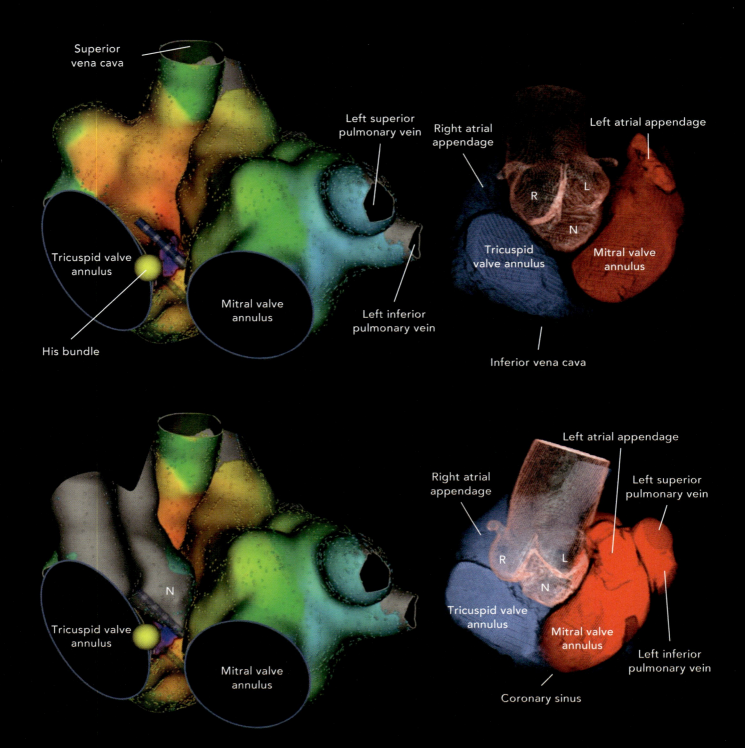

Figure 4-19 *Spotlight:* **Atrial tachycardia ablated from the noncoronary aortic sinus.**

Activation map shows the earliest activation of an atrial tachycardia at the His bundle region. Retrograde aortic mapping shows that the noncoronary aortic sinus is immediately adjacent to both the right- and left-sided para-Hisian regions. Thus, the noncoronary aortic sinus provides a vantage point to both anteroseptal aspects of the right and left atria. Early activation at the para-Hisian region may represent a site of origin that is from the atrial tissue adjacent to the noncoronary aortic sinus or the anteromedial wall of the left atrium.

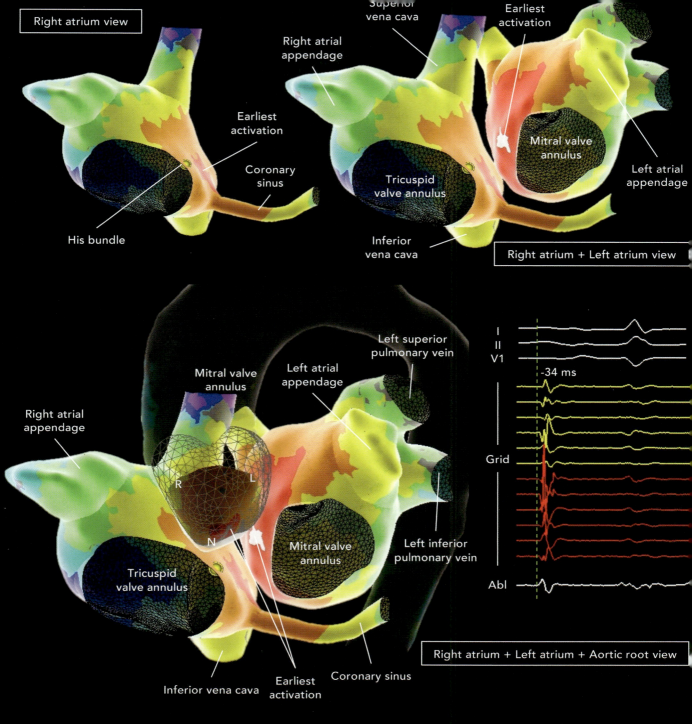

Figure 4-20   Electroanatomic activation mapping of septal atrial tachycardia.

Progressive three-chamber mapping is shown. The initial interpretation suggests right atrial activation i the earliest activation immediately inferior to the His bundle. As the risk of heart block is high, mapping n the left atrium may reveal earlier activation, as seen in this case. With the inclusion of the aortic root he noncoronary aortic sinus timing is the same (−34 ms) as seen within the anteromedial left atrium. Thi ndicates accessibility from two potential vantage points. In this case, successful elimination was achieved rom the left atrium.

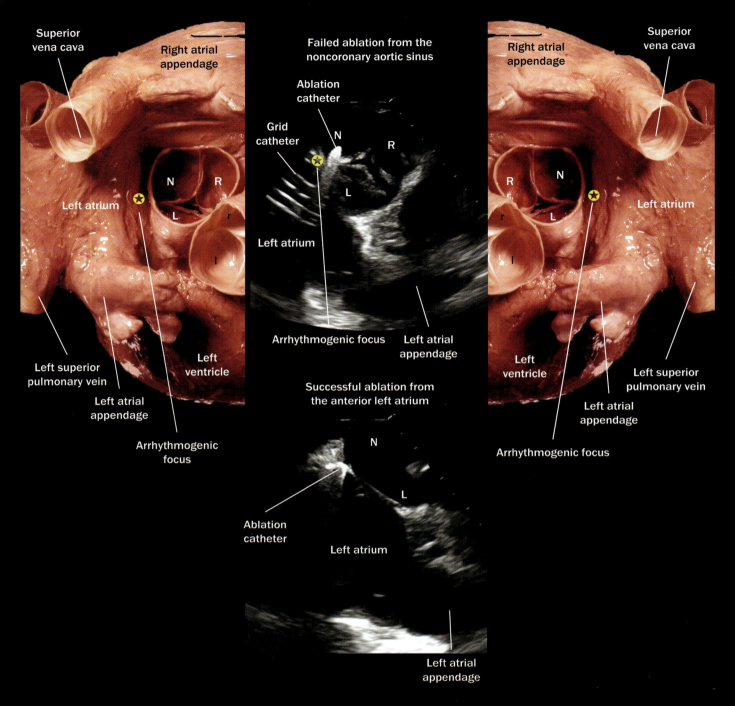

Figure 4-21   Atrial tachycardia originating from the anterior left atrium.

The atrial tachycardia focus (yellow star) was the anterior left atrium adjacent to the noncoronary aortic sinus. A grid catheter within the anterior left atrium is in immediate proximity to the aortic root, where the ablation catheter is placed within the noncoronary aortic sinus (upper). A mirrored anatomical image is shown (left) to enhance the better intracardiac echocardiography interpretation. Initial ablation from the noncoronary aortic sinus failed to eliminate the arrhythmia, but ablation from the anterior left atrium suppressed the focus (bottom).

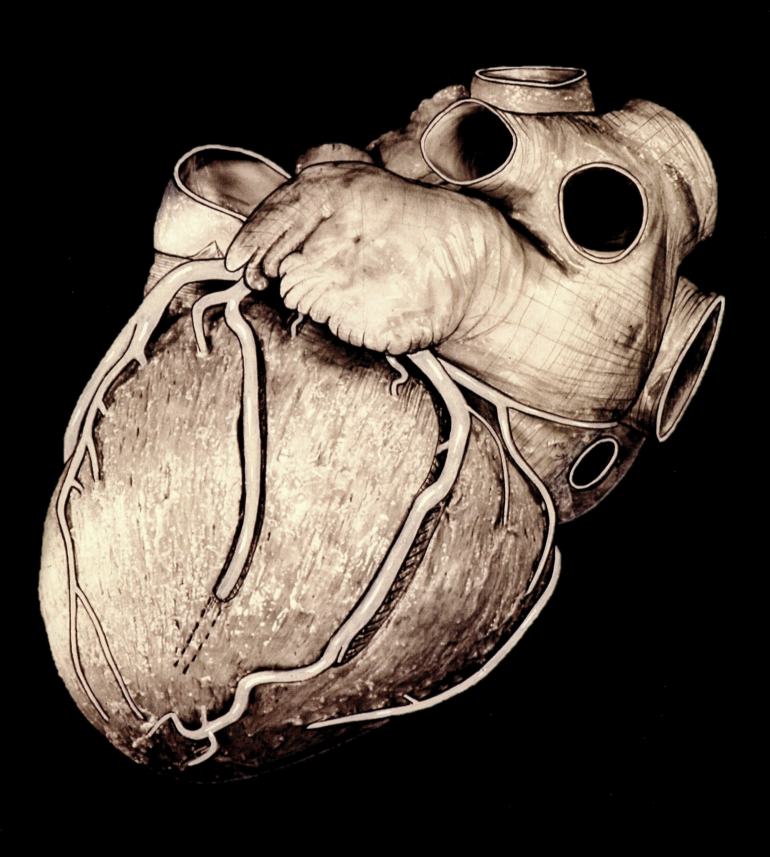

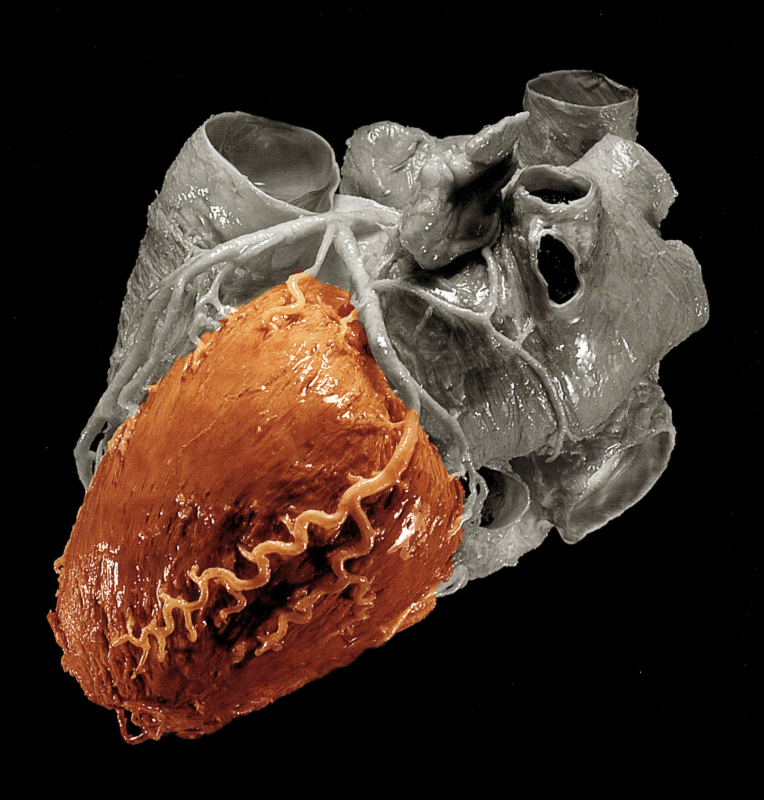

5

The Left Ventricle

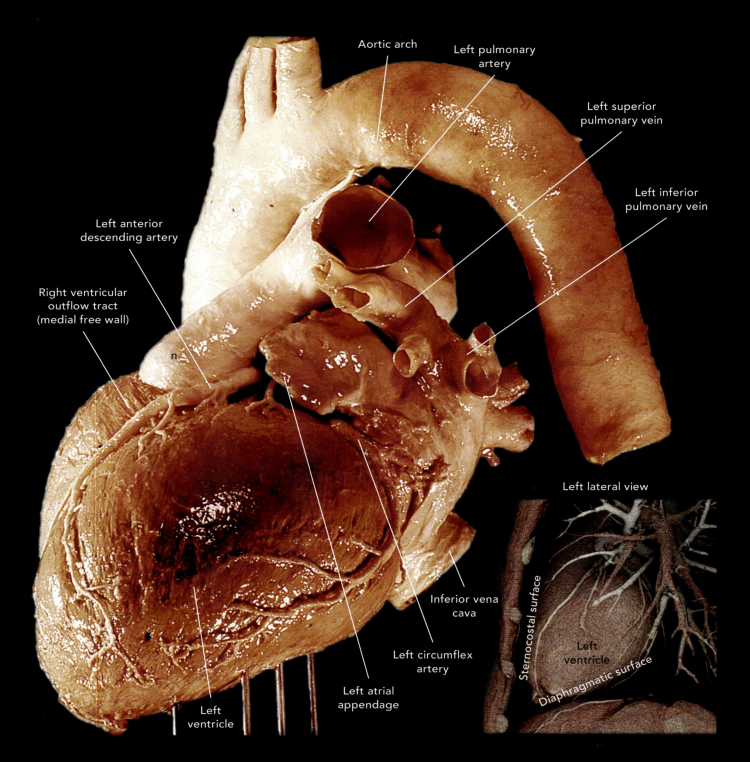

Aortic arch

Left pulmonary artery

Left superior pulmonary vein

Left inferior pulmonary vein

Left anterior descending artery

Right ventricular outflow tract (medial free wall)

n

Left lateral view

Inferior vena cava

Sternocostal surface

Left ventricle

Diaphragmatic surface

Left circumflex artery

Left atrial appendage

Left ventricle

Figure 5-1 **Lateral view of the left ventricle.**

The anterior and inferior wall of the heart corresponds to the sternocostal and diaphragmatic surfaces, respectively. The left anterior descending artery represents the anterior septal boundary of the left ventricle. Behind the boundary, the medial free wall of the right ventricle can be observed. Compared to the ascending aorta, the pulmonary trunk tilts significantly toward the posterior direction. The proximal left coronary artery and the left ventricular summit as its floor cannot be visualized, as they are covered by the left atrial appendage adjacent to the pulmonary trunk.

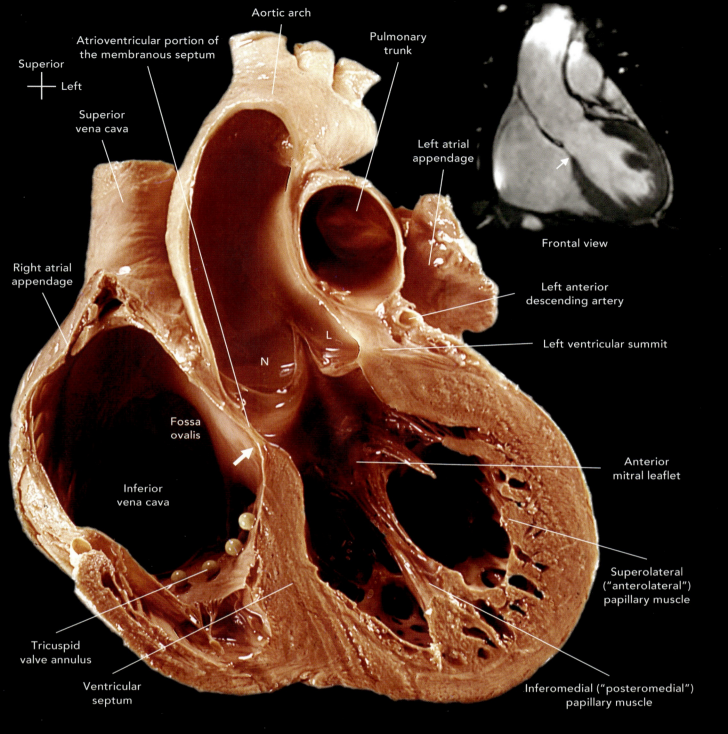

Superior
Left

Aortic arch

Atrioventricular portion of
the membranous septum

Pulmonary
trunk

Superior
vena cava

Left atrial
appendage

Right atrial
appendage

Frontal view

Left anterior
descending artery

Left ventricular summit

N

L

Fossa
ovalis

Anterior
mitral leaflet

Inferior
vena cava

Superolateral
("anterolateral")
papillary muscle

Tricuspid
valve annulus

Ventricular
septum

Inferomedial ("posteromedial")
papillary muscle

Figure 5-2 Coronal section of the left ventricle.

The left ventricular summit represents the highest point of the left ventricle under the proximal left coronary
artery. The left coronary aortic sinus is supported by a beak-shaped myocardium, a thin portion at the
aortic margin of the left ventricular summit. The membranous septum tilts toward the right atrium along
with the tilting of the proximal aorta. This creates an angle between the crest of the ventricular septum.
This angle or dimple (arrows) corresponds to the location of the atrioventricular bundle. An identical
section of cardiac magnetic resonance imaging is shown.

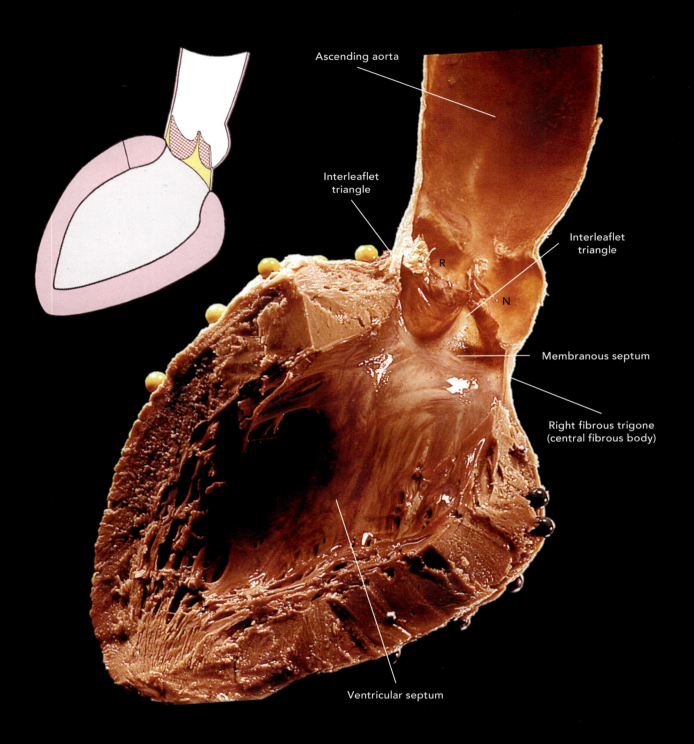

Ascending aorta

Interleaflet triangle

Interleaflet triangle

R

N

Membranous septum

Right fibrous trigone (central fibrous body)

Ventricular septum

Figures 5-3 and 5-4   Septal and lateral left ventricle.

Septal surface of the left ventricle has no papillary muscle, which allows a ventricular transseptal approach from the right ventricle to the left ventricle.[47] Both superolateral and inferomedial papillary muscles do not belong to the ventricular septum, but they are free-wall structures. Specifically, the superolateral and inferomedial papillary muscles are generally located anterolateral and inferior segments of the left ventricle. Thus, the inferolateral segments are the area between the papillary muscles.

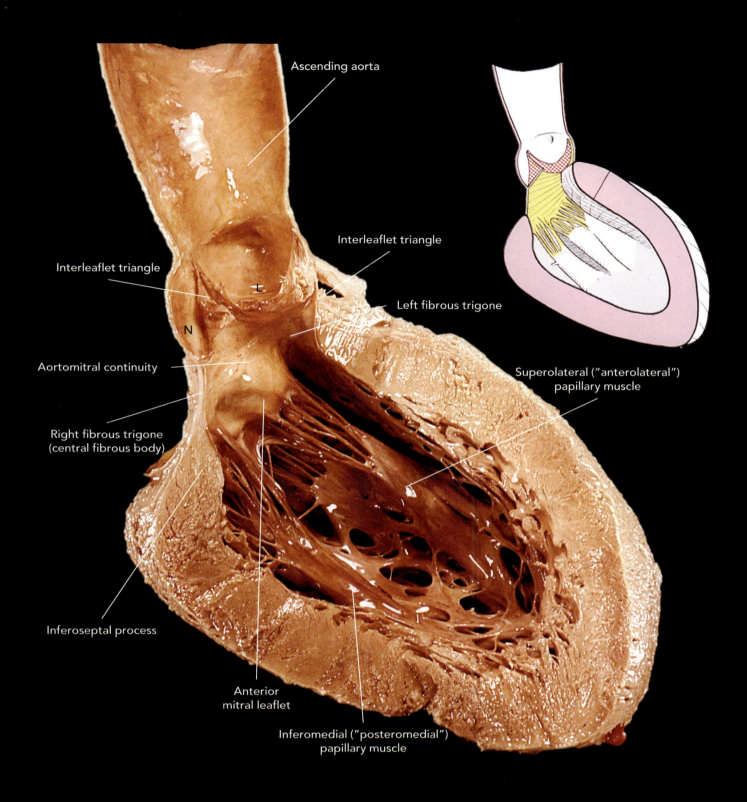

Ascending aorta

Interleaflet triangle

Interleaflet triangle

Left fibrous trigone

Aortomitral continuity

Superolateral ("anterolateral")
papillary muscle

Right fibrous trigone
(central fibrous body)

Inferoseptal process

Anterior
mitral leaflet

Inferomedial ("posteromedial")
papillary muscle

However, in approximately 30%–40% of cases, the intermediate accessory papillary muscle exists between these major papillary muscles, giving the chordae tendineae to the central chordae-free zone of either mitral leaflet.[48] The inferoseptal process is the basal inferoseptal segment, which is actually the free wall facing the anteromedial free wall of the right atrium, intervened by the inferior pyramidal space. In other words, the inferoseptal process faces the floor of the triangle of Koch (Figure 2-26).

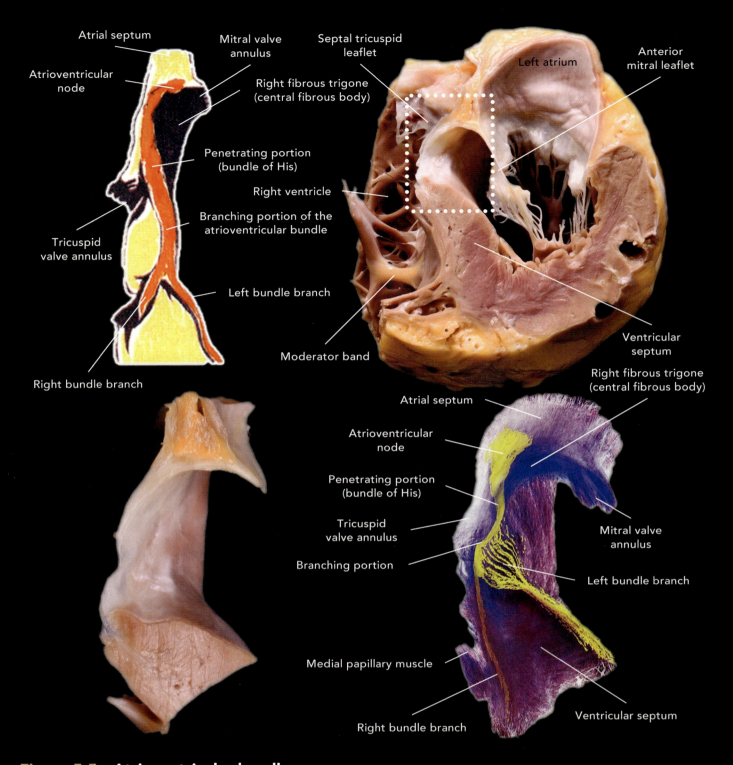

Figure 5-5 Atrioventricular bundle.

Tawara's classic illustration of the atrioventricular bundle[49] is replicated with a digital overlay of the multiple histological sections (Masson-Trichrome) to understand three-dimensionality of his finding in the context of the whole heart.[18] The atrioventricular bundle is colored yellow. The atrioventricular node lies on the right-side central fibrous body, which is penetrated by the His bundle. The proximal origin of the left bundle branch can be appreciated, the width of the branching portion is prominent. The right bundle branch runs beneath the medial papillary muscle.

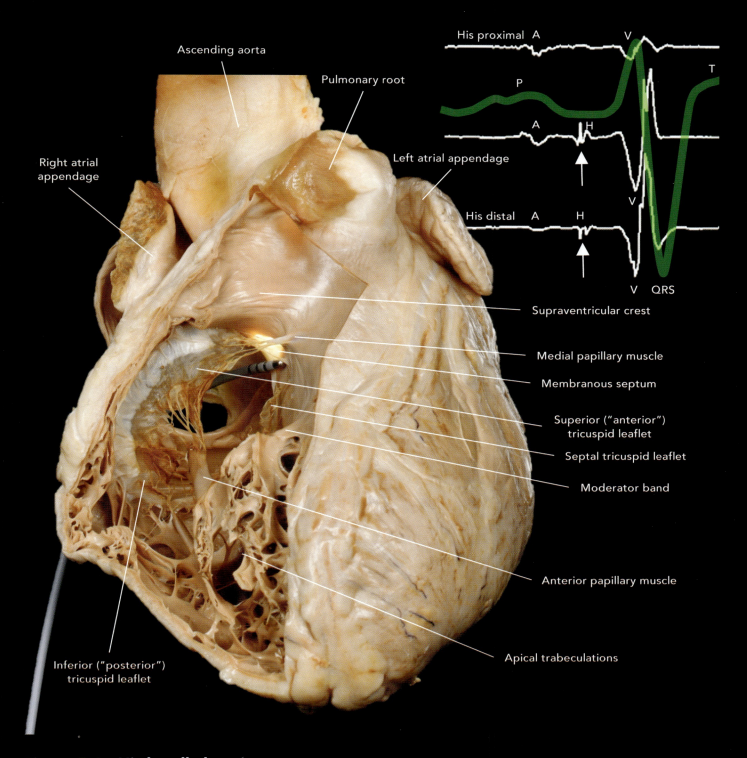

Labels on figure:
- Ascending aorta
- Pulmonary root
- Right atrial appendage
- Left atrial appendage
- His proximal A
- P
- A
- His distal A H
- V
- T
- Supraventricular crest
- Medial papillary muscle
- Membranous septum
- Superior ("anterior") tricuspid leaflet
- Septal tricuspid leaflet
- Moderator band
- Anterior papillary muscle
- Apical trabeculations
- V QRS
- Inferior ("posterior") tricuspid leaflet

Figure 5-6   His bundle location.

The membranous septum (transilluminated) is located at the commissure between the superior and septal tricuspid leaflets. It tilts toward the right atrium along with the tilting of the proximal aorta. This creates an angle between the crest of the ventricular septum. This angle or dimple corresponds to the location of the atrioventricular bundle. His bundle catheter placed exactly at this region along the inferior margin of the membranous septum can record the His and proximal right bundle branch signals (Figure 1-13).

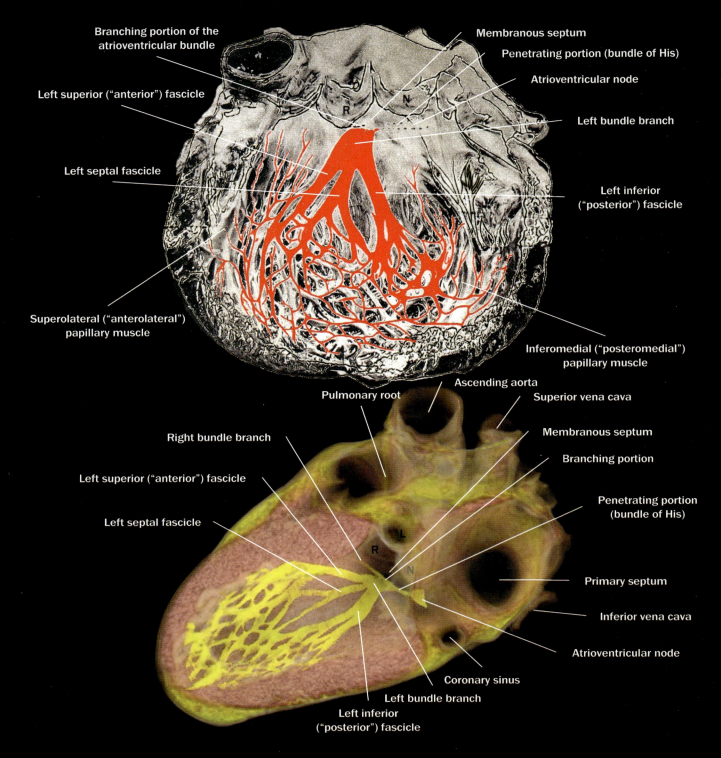

Figure 5-7 Atrioventricular conduction system.

The atrioventricular conduction system illustrated on the opened heart by Tawara,[49] is digitally replicated on the nondistorted heart viewed from the left posterior oblique direction.[50] During intraseptal lead implantation for physiological pacing, the orientation and arborized nature of the left conduction is best appreciated in this left lateral anatomic orientation. After penetration of the right ventricular endocardium, the tip of the pacing lead is advanced in close proximity to the LV septal endocardium. The "anterior" and "posterior" fascicles are oriented superiorly and inferiorly, respectively. Distal left conduction system pacing can yield inferior, indeterminate, and superior electrocardiographic axes depending on which fascicle is captured.

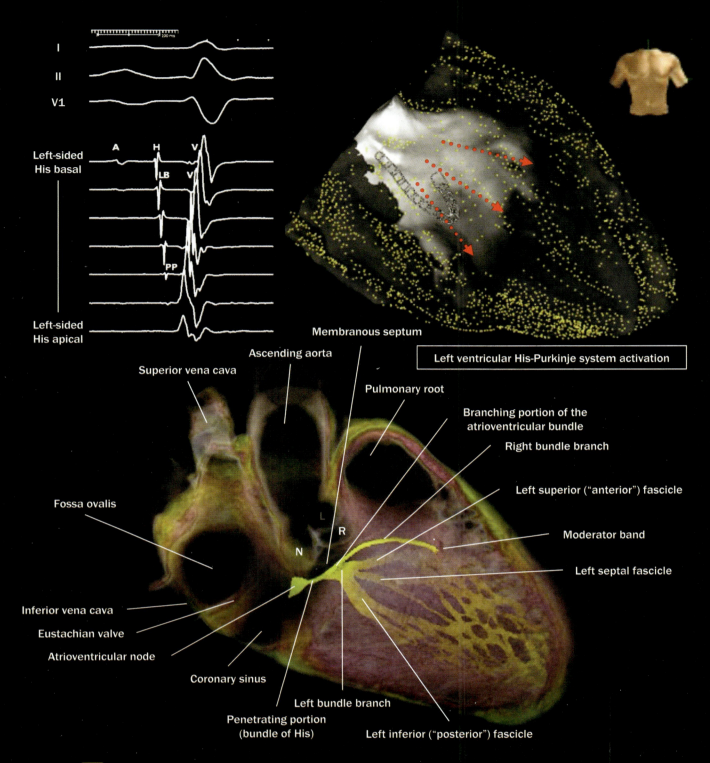

Figure 5-8 ▶ **Physiological His-Purkinje system activation.**

The trifascicular nature of the conduction system is shown with high-density mapping of the left ventricle, with attention to the conduction system signals recorded in the basal septum. There are three broad regions of activation, which are traced with Purkinje potentials that precede the QRS onset. These are consistent with the superior, septal, and inferior fascicles.

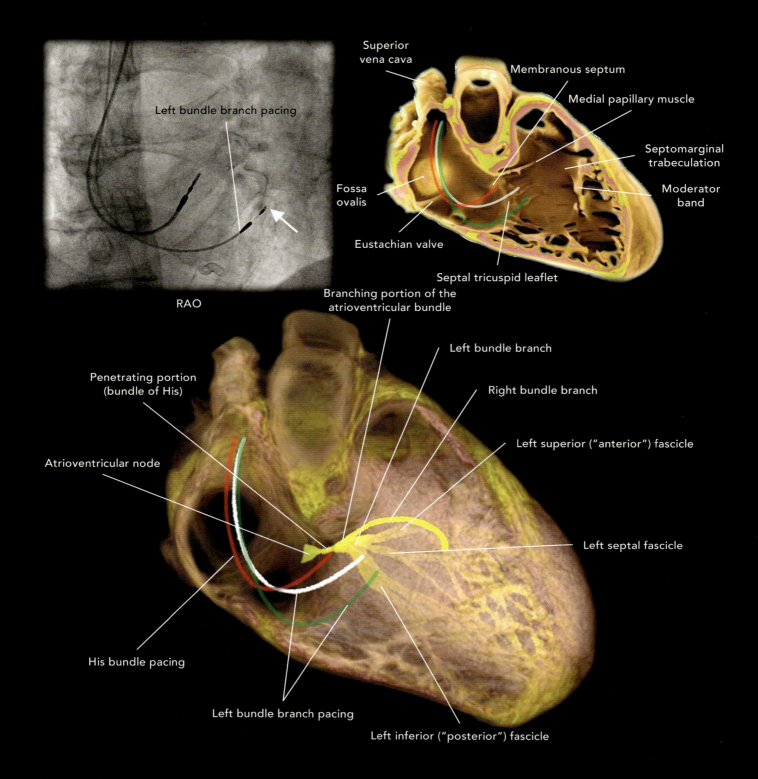

Left bundle branch pacing

RAO

Superior vena cava

Membranous septum

Medial papillary muscle

Septomarginal trabeculation

Moderator band

Fossa ovalis

Eustachian valve

Septal tricuspid leaflet

Branching portion of the atrioventricular bundle

Penetrating portion (bundle of His)

Left bundle branch

Right bundle branch

Left superior ("anterior") fascicle

Atrioventricular node

Left septal fascicle

His bundle pacing

Left bundle branch pacing

Left inferior ("posterior") fascicle

Figures 5-9 and 5-10   Target zones for conduction system pacing.

The His bundle region is predictably at the level of the septal tricuspid valve annulus at the membranous septum between the junction of the noncoronary and right coronary aortic sinuses. This provides a limited anatomic target zone for lead fixation. In contrast, the left bundle branch area, and fascicular divisions are arborized and provide a wide target zone for lead fixation into the left ventricular endocardial side of the ventricular septum. Consider the course of the septal branches (Figure 3-22).

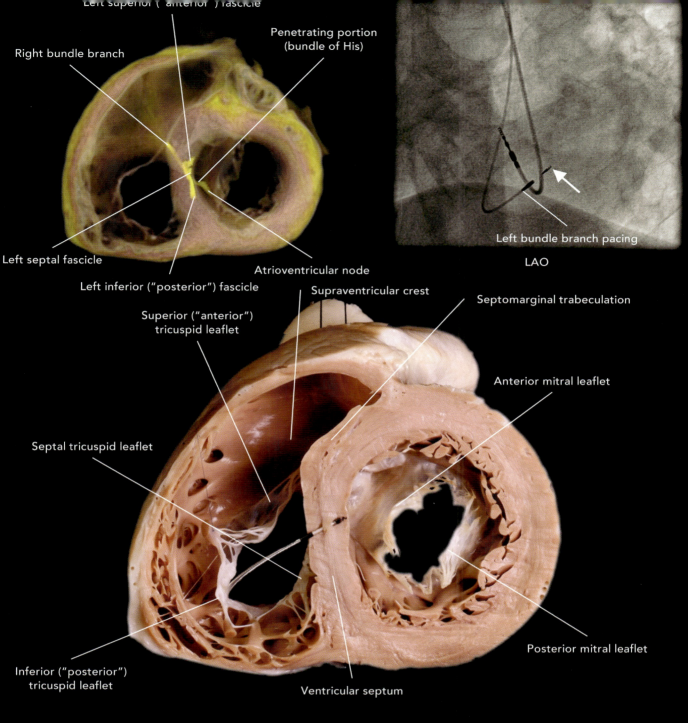

Left superior ("anterior") fascicle

Right bundle branch

Penetrating portion (bundle of His)

Left septal fascicle

Left inferior ("posterior") fascicle

Atrioventricular node

Left bundle branch pacing

LAO

Supraventricular crest

Septomarginal trabeculation

Superior ("anterior") tricuspid leaflet

Anterior mitral leaflet

Septal tricuspid leaflet

Inferior ("posterior") tricuspid leaflet

Ventricular septum

Posterior mitral leaflet

As the His bundle pacing is performed at the commissure, there is a minimal risk of fixing the septal tricuspid leaflet and inducing lead-related exacerbation of tricuspid regurgitation.[23] As the ventricular septum is a convex-shaped structure, perpendicular placement of the lead targeting the septal and inferior fascicle is technically easier within the inferoseptal segment than targeting the superior fascicle distributing within the anteroseptal segment.

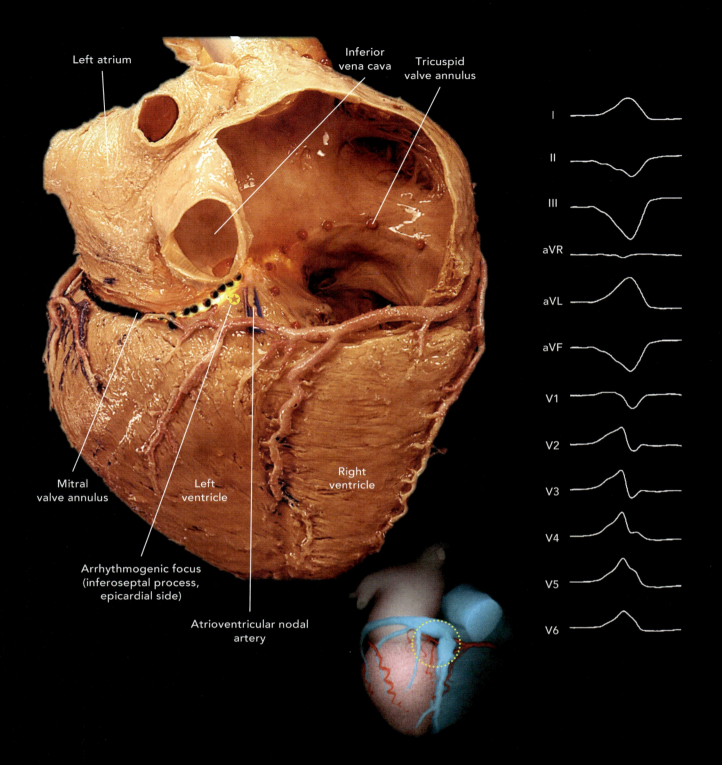

Left atrium

Inferior vena cava

Tricuspid valve annulus

I

II

III

aVR

aVL

aVF

V1

V2

V3

V4

V5

V6

Mitral valve annulus

Left ventricle

Right ventricle

Arrhythmogenic focus
(inferoseptal process,
epicardial side)

Atrioventricular nodal
artery

Figure 5-11   **Ventricular arrhythmia from the crux of the heart.**

The crux of the heart represents the inferior intersection between all four chambers (Figure 2-34), corresponding to the epicardial side of the inferoseptal process.[51] The ventricular arrhythmias from this epicardial area show indeterminate bundle branch morphology with abrupt R-wave transition from V1 to V2 with a left superior axis.[52] The posteromedial left atrial ganglionated plexus (Figure 2-13) located in this region around the coronary sinus orifice[11] is a target for neuromodulation in patients with vagally mediated atrioventricular block.

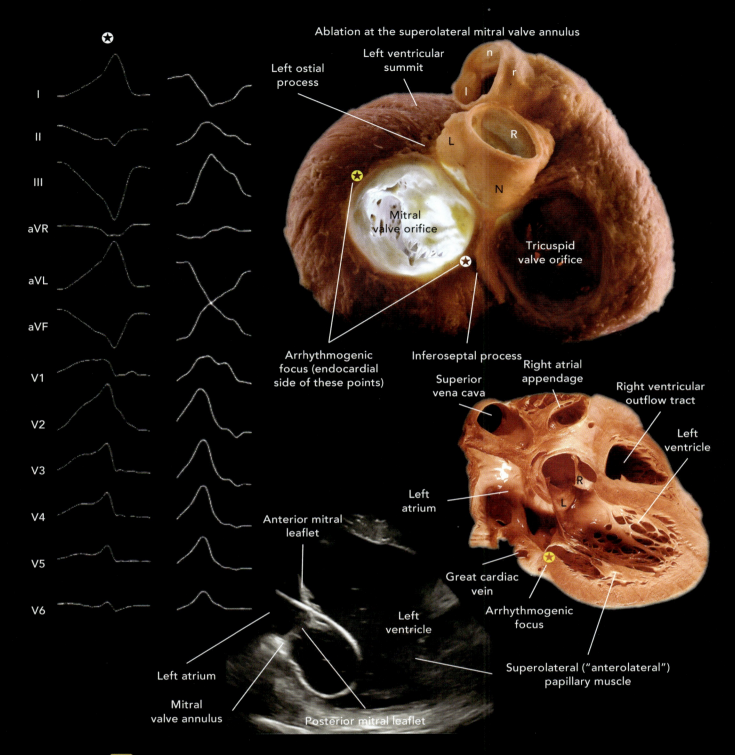

Ablation at the superolateral mitral valve annulus

Left ventricular
summit

Left ostial
process

Mitral
valve orifice

Tricuspid
valve orifice

Arrhythmogenic
focus (endocardial
side of these points)

Inferoseptal process

Superior
vena cava

Right atrial
appendage

Right ventricular
outflow tract

Left
ventricle

Left
atrium

Great cardiac
vein

Arrhythmogenic
focus

Superolateral ("anterolateral")
papillary muscle

Anterior mitral
leaflet

Left
ventricle

Left atrium

Mitral
valve annulus

Posterior mitral leaflet

Figure 5-12 ▶ Mitral annular ventricular arrhythmia.

Isthmuses that run parallel to the mitral valve annulus can be paired with opposite QRS morphology[53] that emerges from the superolateral annulus (R-wave concordance with inferior axis—yellow star) and the inferoseptal annulus (R-wave concordance with left superior axis—white star). Both retrograde and antegrade U-turn approaches can access the subvalvular annulus, and optimal catheter location can be confirmed with intracardiac echocardiography. The inferoseptal annulus corresponds to the endocardial side of the inferoseptal process.[19, 23, 51, 54]

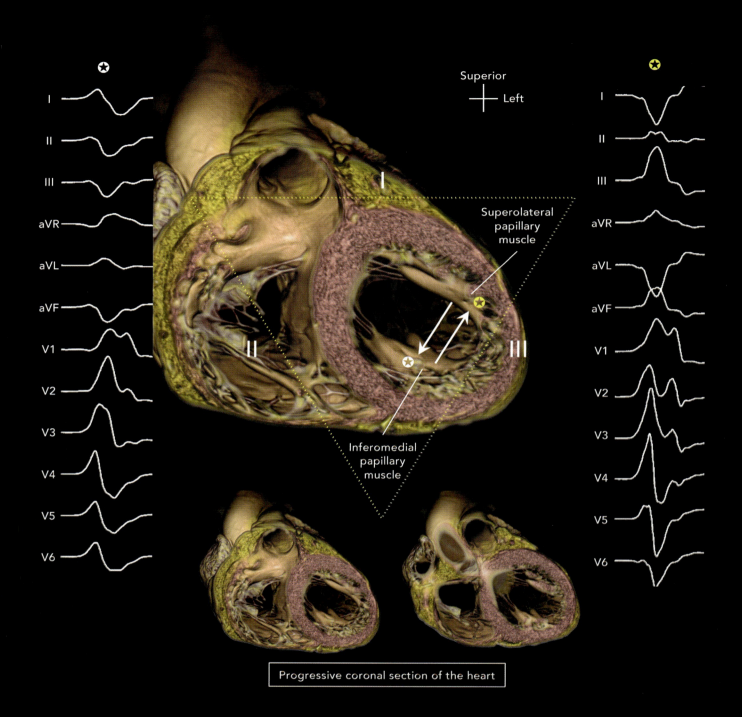

Progressive coronal section of the heart

Figures 5-13 and 5-14 Left ventricular papillary muscles.

The superolateral ("anterolateral") and inferomedial ("posteromedial") papillary muscles are important sites of ventricular arrhythmias,[55, 56] namely premature ventricular contractions, and less commonly monomorphic ventricular tachycardia. They have opposite QRS polarities along the axis of lead III as shown by the triangulation shown on the coronal section of the left ventricle cut at the papillary muscle level. An inferomedial site of origin (white star) yields a superior axis with lead III S > lead II S, and a superolateral site of origin (yellow star) yields an inferior axis with lead III R > lead II R. There is an important overlap between fascicular ventricular arrhythmia with papillary muscle arrhythmias.[57] In general, wider QRS and atypical right bundle branch block patterns are suggestive of papillary muscle origin.

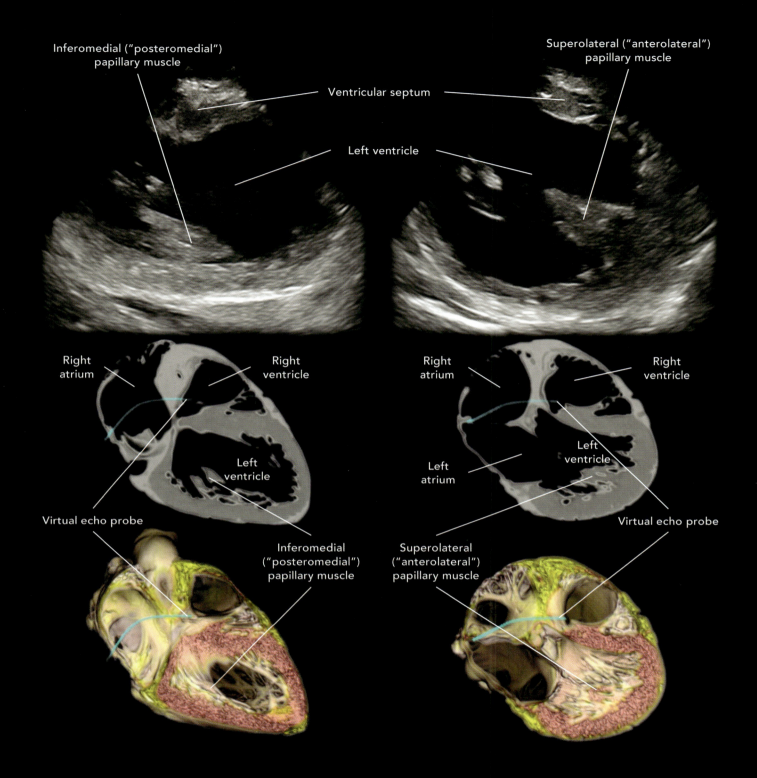

The base of the papillary muscle must be differentiated from the tip of the papillary muscle with the use of intracardiac echocardiography during mapping. It greatly facilitates the ability to map and record around the entire papillary muscle as well as monitor lesion formation during radiofrequency energy delivery. After anterior flexion into the right ventricle, clockwise rotation visualizes the inferoseptal papillary muscle first after the ventricular septum. With additional clockwise movement, a more superior portion of the left ventricle is seen with the emergence of the superolateral papillary muscle.

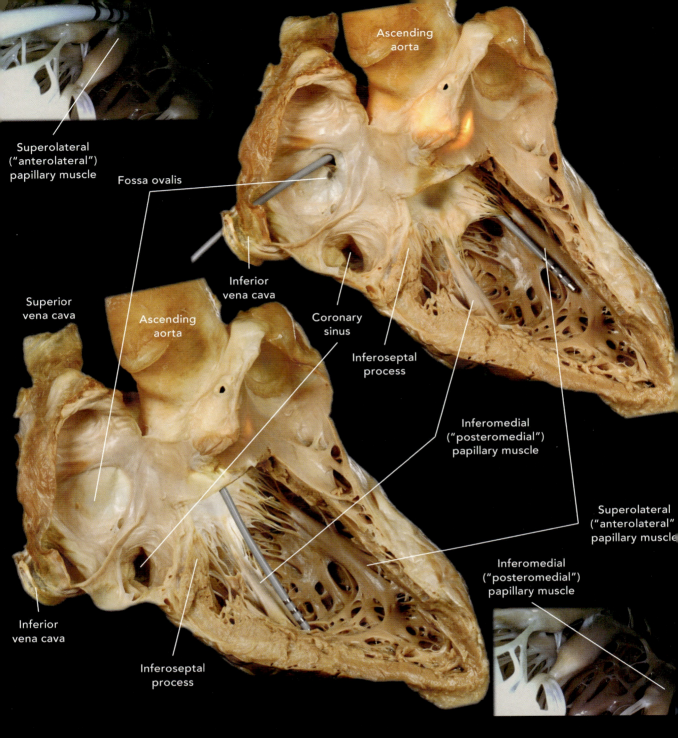

Figure 5-15 **Mapping of the papillary muscles.**

With a retroaortic approach, the catheter directs toward the base of the inferomedial papillary musc[le] corresponding to the mid-inferolateral wall of the left ventricle. This is because of the physiological aort[ic] [t]o-left ventricular axial angulation. With a transseptal approach, the catheter runs along the superolate[ral] [p]apillary muscle. Appreciating this anatomical relationship is important to select optimal approach [f]or simple and effective mapping and ablation of each papillary muscle as a complicated left ventricu[lar] [m]anipulation has a risk of entrapment/entanglement.

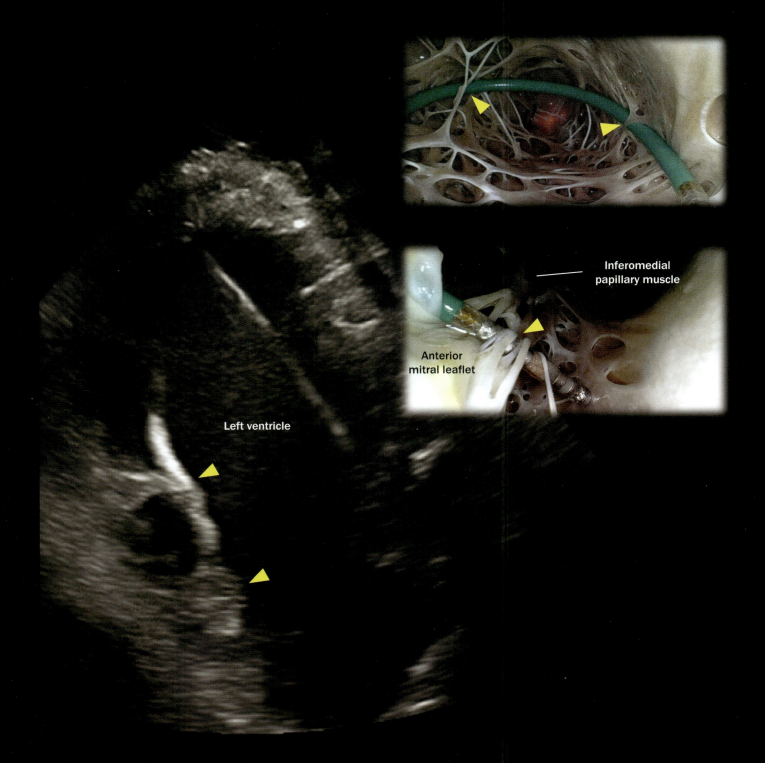

Left ventricle

Inferomedial
papillary muscle

Anterior
mitral leaflet

Figure 5-16 ▶ *Spotlight:* **Catheter entrapment within the left ventricle.**

The papillary muscles, chordae tendineae, and multi-layered fine trabeculations are important intracavitary structures that impede catheter manipulation. Catheters may become entrapped by or entangled with these structures (arrowheads), especially during U-turned and torqued approach. Importantly, additional torquing and forced retraction may worsen the entanglement. The most optimal method is the careful advancement with counter torquing followed by an attempt to straighten the catheter while advancing a long sheath into the left ventricle, akin to a lead extraction.

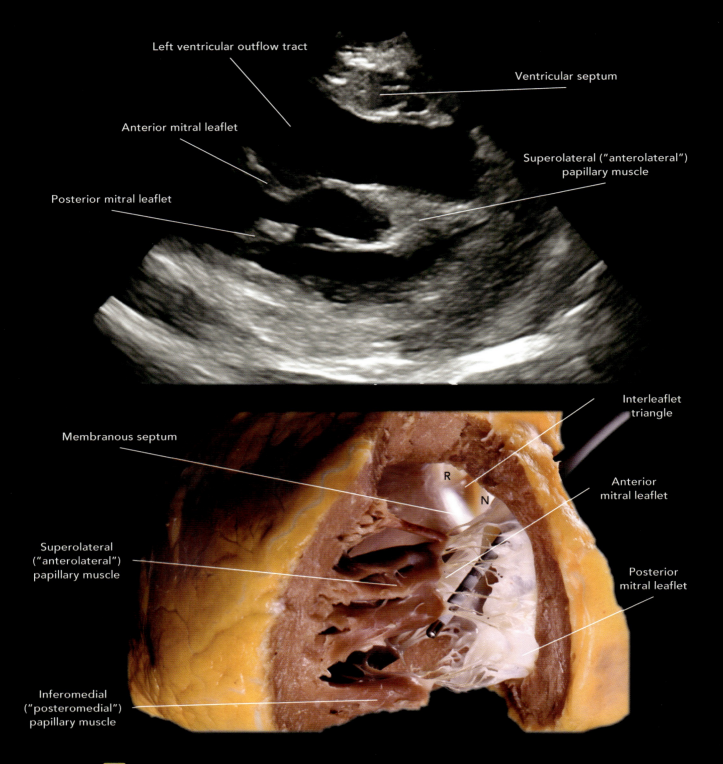

Figure 5-17 ▶ **Superolateral papillary muscle.**

The superolateral papillary muscle in these images appears as multiple heads with separate bands of chordal attachments. Visualization on intracardiac echocardiography is achieved with clockwise rotation from the more inferiorly located inferomedial papillary muscle. Transseptal access readily provides access to this region, and counterclockwise rotation of the sheath is useful to navigate the left ventricle toward the apical and septal aspects of the left ventricle.

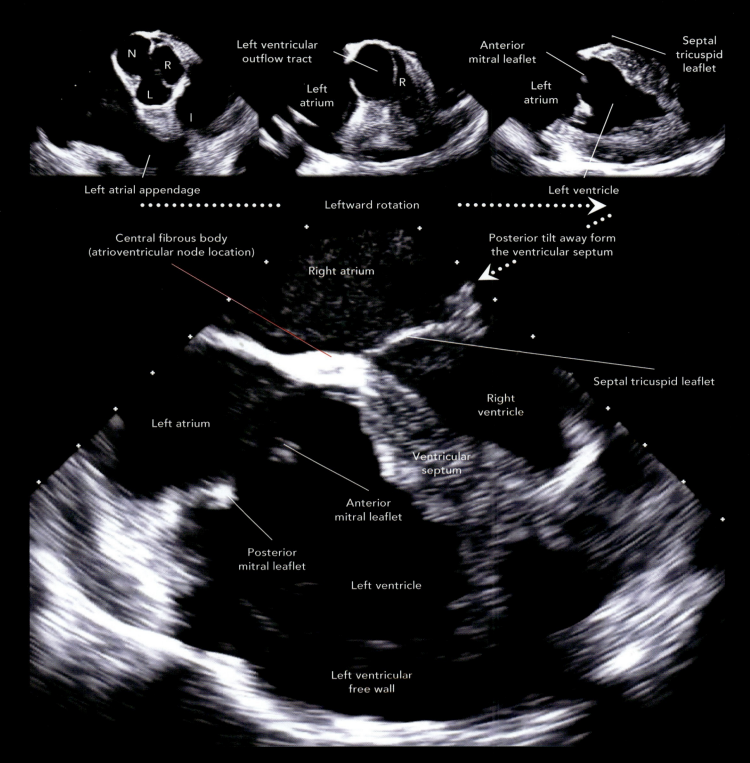

Figure 5-18 ▶ **Four-chamber view of the heart on intracardiac echocardiography.**

This view can be achieved by advancing the probe into the right ventricle with clockwise torque until the aortic valve is seen in short-axis view. From this position, a posterior tilt brings the heart into view of the septum below the aortic valve. This view is optimal to assess septal substrate as the routine left ventricular views from the right ventricle are too close to the septum. Biventricular mapping or bipolar ablation can be optimized in this view to visualize both right and left sides of the septum (Figure 5-20).

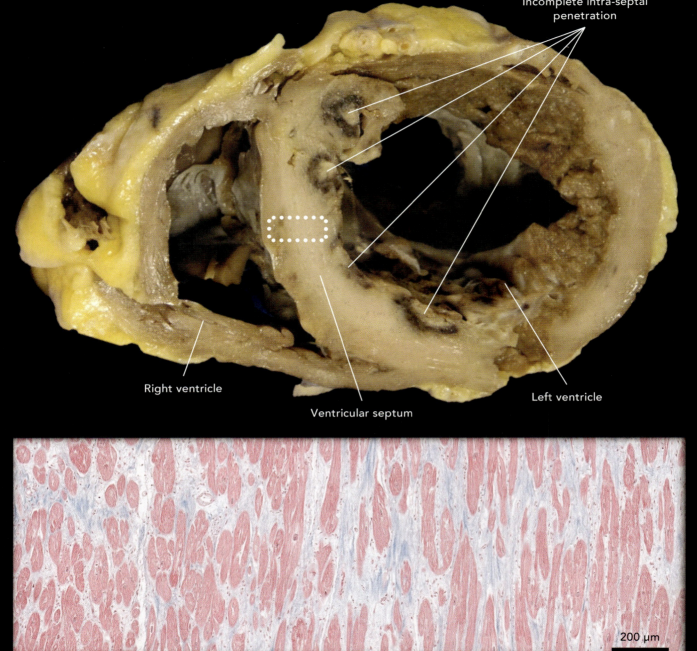

Figure 5-19 **Mid-myocardial septal scar substrate.**

Examination of explanted heart after cardiac transplantation in a patient with multiple prior ablations on the left-sided ventricular septum shows that the radiofrequency lesions incompletely penetrate the septum and mid-myocardium. The nontransmural nature of radiofrequency lesions highlights the difficulty in addressing septal substrates, particularly those with mid-myocardial fibrosis, which is common in genetic cardiomyopathies. Bottom panel shows mid-myocardial interstitial fibrosis.

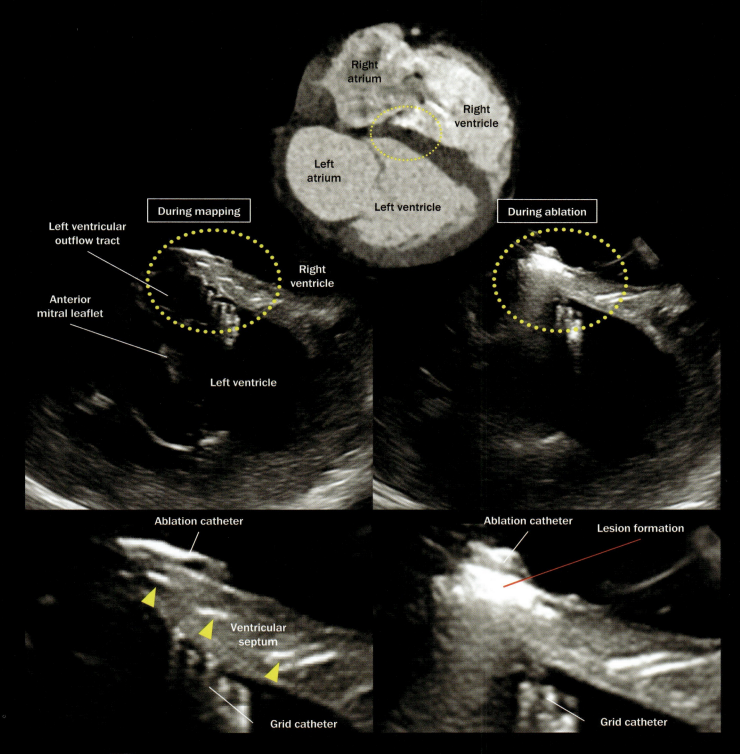

Figure 5-20 ▶ **Biventricular mapping and ablation of intraseptal substrate.**

A sandwich mapping approach of the septum can be visualized using intracardiac echocardiography. Increased echogenicity (arrowheads) may indicate mid-septal substrate. In these images, a grid catheter is placed via transseptal approach on the left-sided ventricular septum, and the ablation catheter is parallel to the right-sided ventricular septum. Lesion formation during radiofrequency application can be monitored by increased echogenicity but results in incomplete penetration across the ventricular septum.

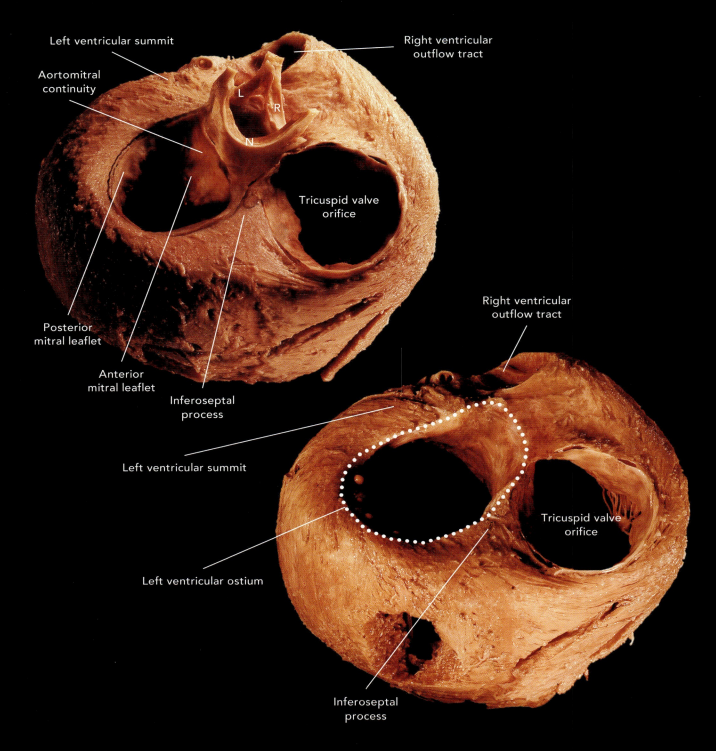

Figure 5-21 **Left ventricular ostium.**

In contrast to the right ventricle, the atrioventricular and semilunar arterial valves are not separated by the ventricular muscle but connected with the fibrous curtain of the aortomitral continuity. Thus, when the mitral-aortic valve complex is removed without removing the ventricular myocardium, an intact single orifice (white dotted line) can be observed at the base of the left ventricle, referred to as the left ventricular ostium. The left ventricular summit and inferoseptal process are located superior and inferoseptal to the left ventricular ostium, respectively.

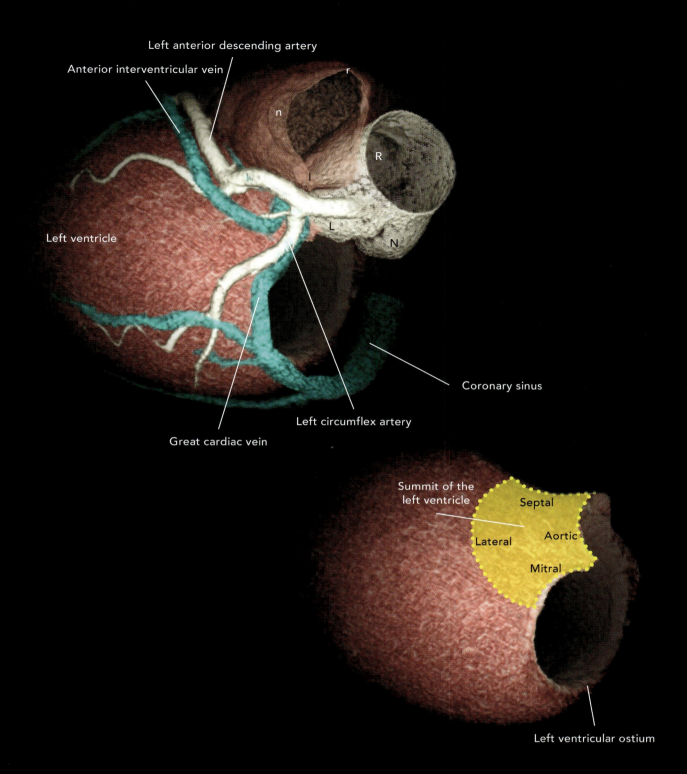

Left anterior descending artery

Anterior interventricular vein

r

n

R

I

L

N

Left ventricle

Coronary sinus

Great cardiac vein

Left circumflex artery

Summit of the
left ventricle

Septal

Aortic

Lateral

Mitral

Left ventricular ostium

Figure 5-22 Left ventricular summit.

The heart is viewed from the cranial direction. Progressive dissection demonstrates the summit of the left ventricle and its four margins.[58] The septal margin corresponds to the superior attachment of the right ventricle, facing to the posterior free wall of the infundibulum. The aortic margin faces the left coronary aortic sinus and the interleaflet triangle between the right and left coronary aortic sinuses. The mitral margin faces the mitral valve annulus. No anatomical counterpart is found at the lateral margin.

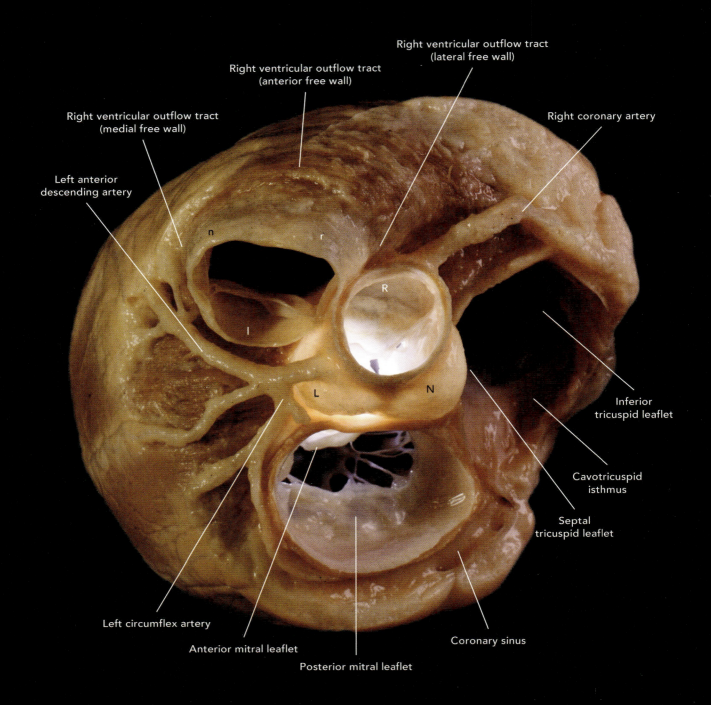

Right ventricular outflow tract
(medial free wall)

Right ventricular outflow tract
(anterior free wall)

Right ventricular outflow tract
(lateral free wall)

Right coronary artery

Left anterior
descending artery

n   r

R

Inferior
tricuspid leaflet

L   N

Cavotricuspid
isthmus

Septal
tricuspid leaflet

Left circumflex artery

Anterior mitral leaflet

Posterior mitral leaflet

Coronary sinus

Figures 5-23 and 5-24   Progressive dissection of the pulmonary root at the level of the subpulmonary infundibulum.

The heart is viewed from the right anterior oblique and cranial direction from the ascending aorta.

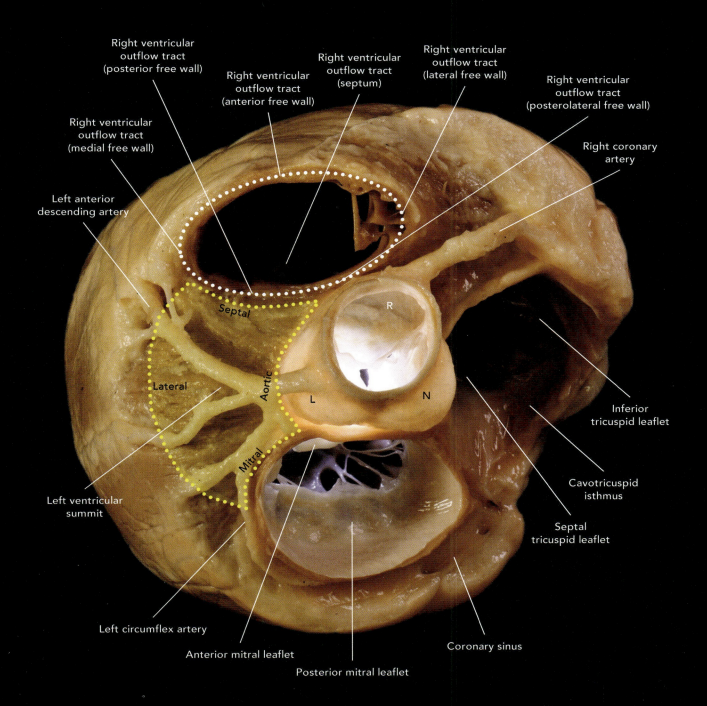

Right ventricular outflow tract (posterior free wall)

Right ventricular outflow tract (anterior free wall)

Right ventricular outflow tract (septum)

Right ventricular outflow tract (lateral free wall)

Right ventricular outflow tract (posterolateral free wall)

Right ventricular outflow tract (medial free wall)

Right coronary artery

Left anterior descending artery

Septal

R

Lateral

Aortic

L

N

Inferior tricuspid leaflet

Mitral

Cavotricuspid isthmus

Left ventricular summit

Septal tricuspid leaflet

Left circumflex artery

Coronary sinus

Anterior mitral leaflet

Posterior mitral leaflet

The pulmonary root is removed at the level of the subpulmonary infundibulum (distal right ventricular outflow tract). The relationship between the free-standing subpulmonary infundibulum and the summit of the left ventricle is readily appreciated. Also, six segments of the right ventricular outflow tract (Figure 3-26) are recognized. Comprehensive topographic understanding of each margin and segment is important to understand electrocardiography and to select an appropriate approach to ablate ventricular arrhythmias originating from these most complicated regions.

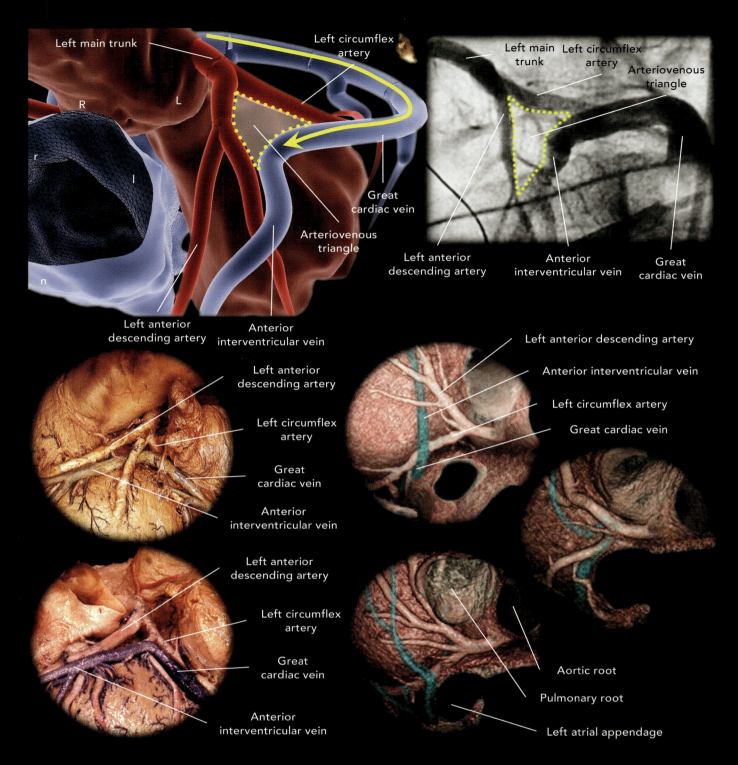

Figure 5-25 Arteriovenous triangle.

The "inaccessible" area[59] is identical to the arteriovenous triangle created by the proximal left anterior descending artery, left circumflex artery, and the anterior interventricular vein, and only the part of the left ventricular summit. This region is only accessible through direct surgical or percutaneous epicardial approaches. Simultaneous coronary angiography and coronary sinus venography (upper right) illustrate the arteriovenous triangle. The arteriovenous relationship is markedly variable (bottom panels).

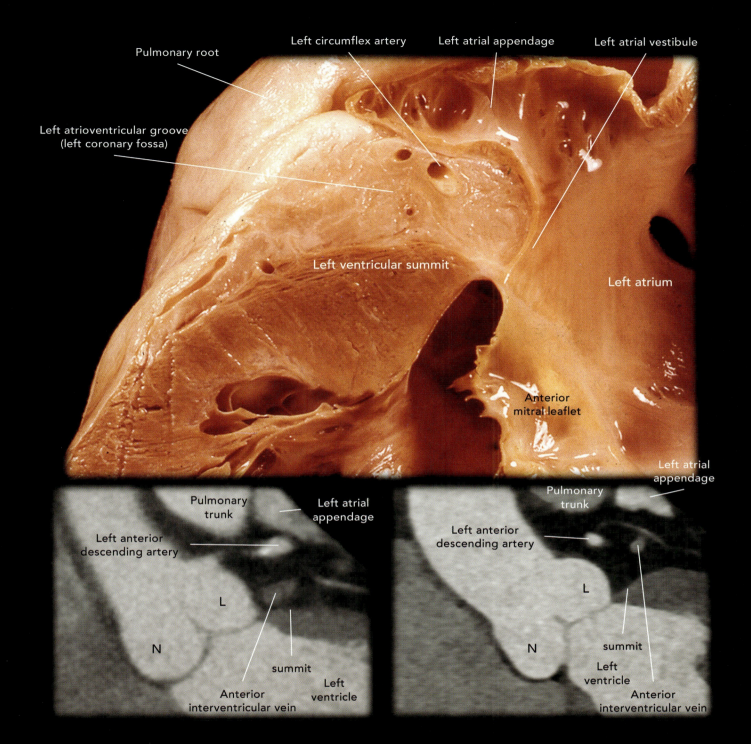

Pulmonary root

Left circumflex artery

Left atrial appendage

Left atrial vestibule

Left atrioventricular groove
(left coronary fossa)

Left ventricular summit

Left atrium

Anterior
mitral leaflet

Left atrial
appendage

Pulmonary
trunk

Left atrial
appendage

Left anterior
descending artery

Pulmonary
trunk

Left anterior
descending artery

L

L

N

N

summit

summit

Anterior
interventricular vein

Left
ventricle

Left
ventricle

Anterior
interventricular vein

Figure 5-26   Left coronary fossa.

The compartment filled with thick epicardial fat is referred to as the left coronary fossa (Figure 4-2) between the left atrial appendage and the left ventricular summit. It involves the proximal left coronary artery, great cardiac vein, and anterior interventricular vein. The thickness of the fat and the relative location of the coronary vessels within the fat are variable (bottom panels). This indicates the utility and feasibility of preprocedural evaluation of coronary vessels using cardiac computed tomography. Note the beak-shaped appearance of the myocardium supporting the left coronary aortic sinus.

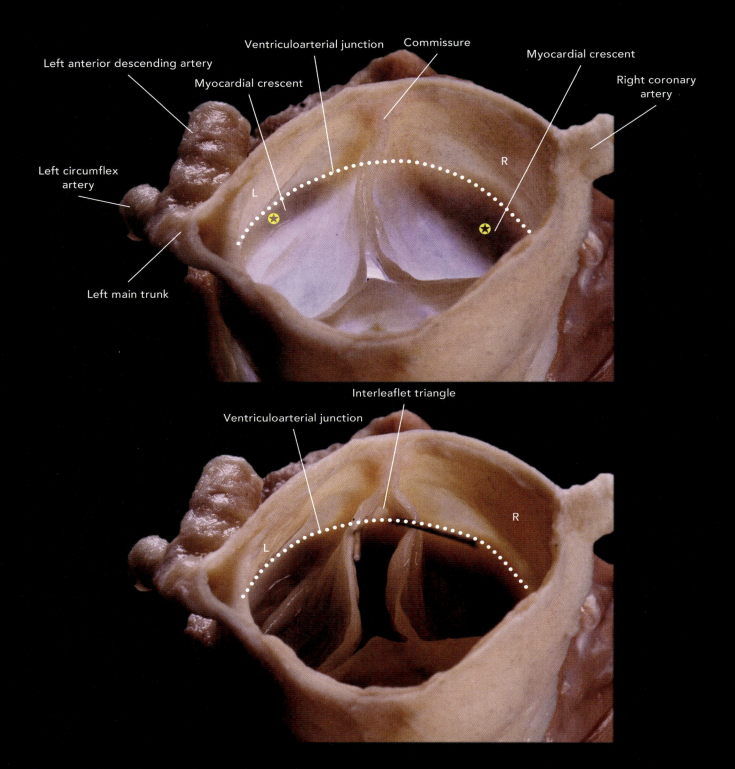

Figure 5-27 Ventriculoarterial junction.

The ventriculoarterial junction represents the left ventricular ostium supporting the aortic root. The right coronary aortic sinus and the anterior half of the left coronary aortic sinus are directly supported (yellow stars, myocardial crescents), whereas the ventriculoarterial junction is located distal to the semilunar hinge line of each leaflet. However, it is located proximal to the interleaflet triangle, supporting its subvalvular base.[60] The ventriculoarterial junction supporting the left coronary aortic sinus and interleaflet triangle corresponds to the aortic margin of the left ventricular summit (Figure 5-28).

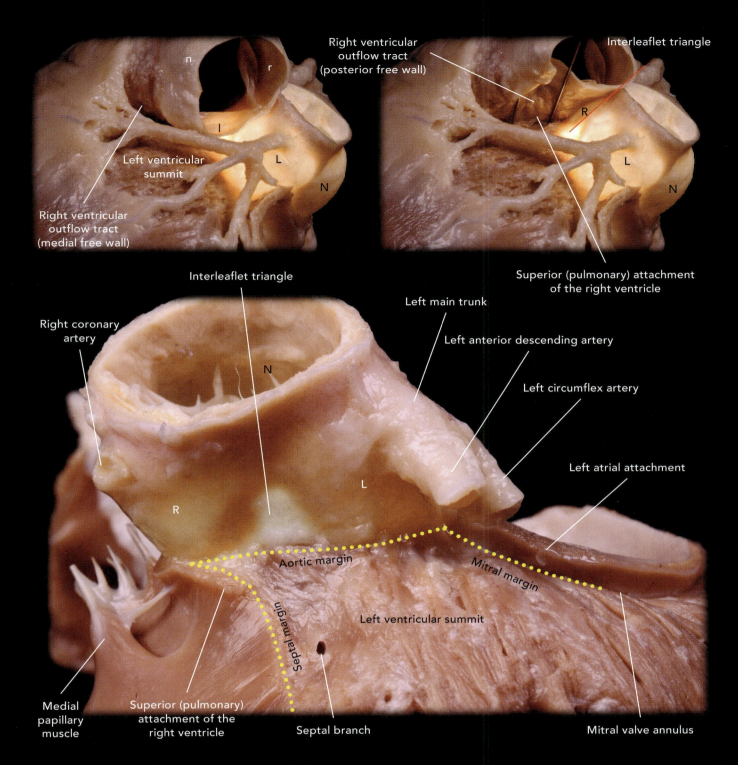

Right ventricular outflow tract (posterior free wall)

Interleaflet triangle

n   r

Left ventricular summit

I

L

N

Right ventricular outflow tract (medial free wall)

R

L

N

Superior (pulmonary) attachment of the right ventricle

Interleaflet triangle

Left main trunk

Left anterior descending artery

Left circumflex artery

Right coronary artery

N

L

R

Left atrial attachment

Aortic margin

Mitral margin

Septal margin

Left ventricular summit

Mitral valve annulus

Medial papillary muscle

Superior (pulmonary) attachment of the right ventricle

Septal branch

Figure 5-28   Interleaflet triangle.

There are three interleaflet triangles in the aortic root. Only the one between the right and left coronary aortic sinuses is supported by the ventricular muscle of the left ventricular ostium, corresponding to the ventriculoarterial junction/aortic margin of the left ventricular summit. As the interleaflet triangle is the subvalvular structure, and only the base of the triangle is supported by the myocardium, a subvalvular approach is necessary to target a ventricular arrhythmia related to this region.[60]

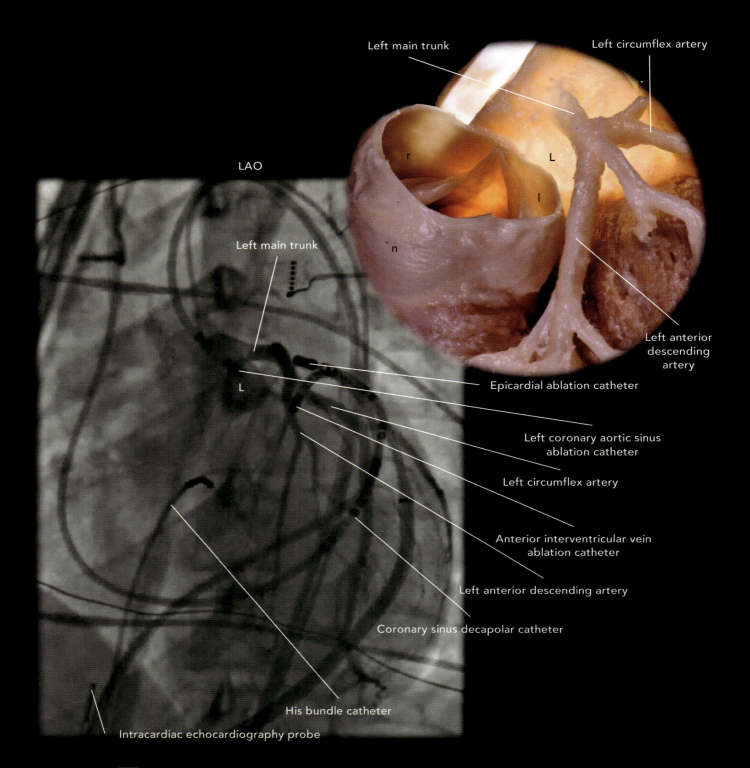

Figure 5-29 ▶ **Mapping the left ventricular ostium and left main trunk.**

Left ventricular summit arrhythmias arise immediately under the left main trunk. Mapping performed around this area can be achieved through multiple vantage points. In this fluoroscopic image, the catheters are mapping the region around the left main trunk: 1) left coronary aortic sinus through a retrograde approach; 2) epicardial left ventricle through percutaneous subxiphoid access; and 3) the junction between the great cardiac vein and anterior interventricular vein through the coronary sinus.

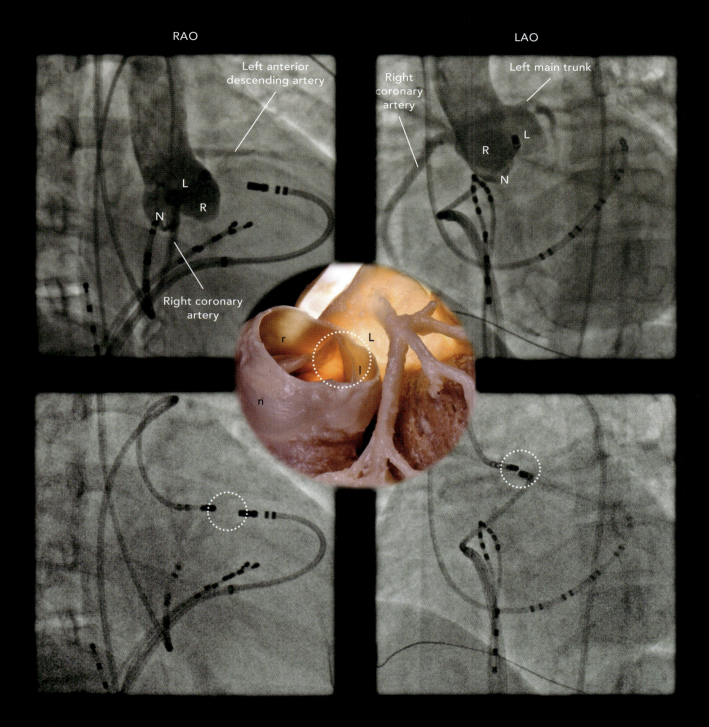

Figure 5-30 Mapping around the interleaflet triangle.

Fluoroscopic images show mapping around the interleaflet triangle between the right and left coronary aortic sinuses. The interleaflet is adjacent to the interleaflet triangle between the right and left adjacent pulmonary sinus. A retroaortic catheter and a sigmoid-shaped antegrade catheter placed at the pulmonary root confirm proximity of both interleaflet triangles.

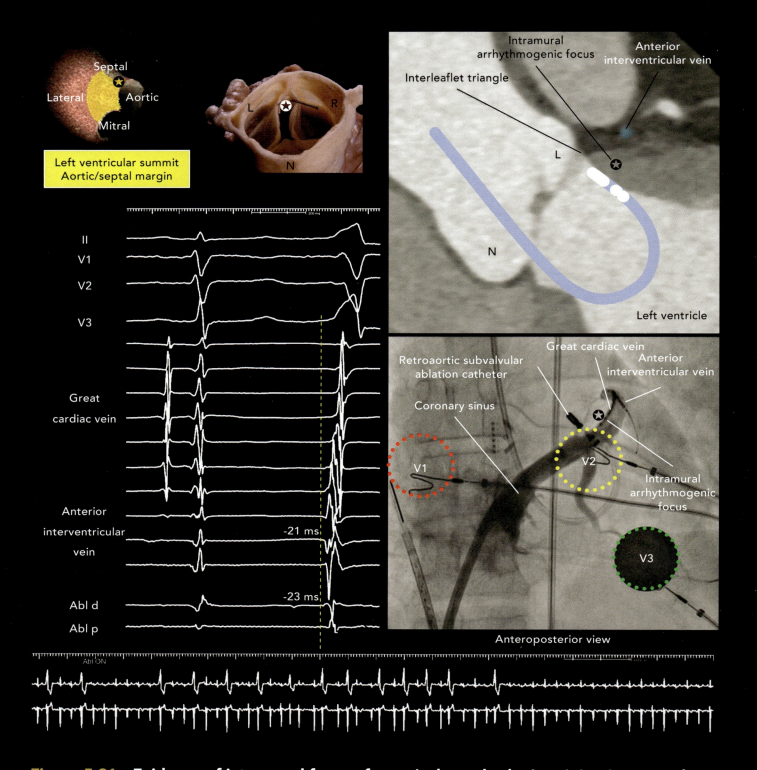

Figure 5-31 **Evidence of intramural focus of ventricular arrhythmia originating near the interleaflet triangle.**

Intramural focus is defined by broad activation, earliest activation <30 ms, and equal timing from endocardial and epicardial recordings. The earliest activation is –21 ms from the epicardium through the anterior interventricular vein and –23 ms from the base of the interleaflet triangle. Both electrograms are far-field in nature, indicating an earlier site within the mid-myocardial planes. Endocardial ablation eliminated the arrhythmia after 14 ms, also supporting an intramural origin. Note the abrupt V3 transition.[61]

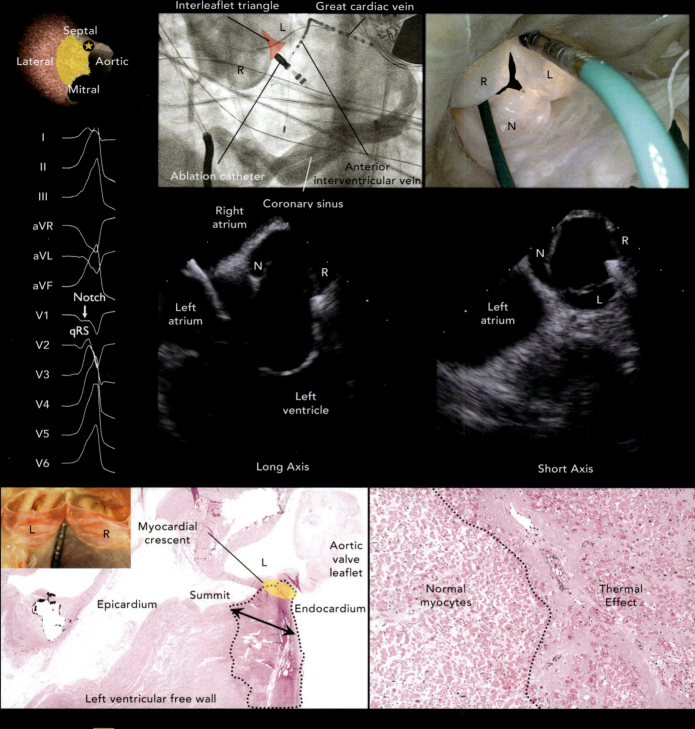

Figure 5-32 ▶ *Spotlight:* **Ventricular arrhythmia ablated from interleaflet triangle vantage point.**

Long-axis views of the catheter profile via transseptal approach show that the catheter is at the level of the ventriculoarterial junction. Short-axis view confirms the interleaflet location (middle panels). The upper panels show the retroaortic U-turn approach. The bottom panels show ex-vivo application of the radiofrequency energy to the base of the interleaflet triangle with partially transmural effect confirmed by histology. A characteristic W or notch pattern in V1 is a signature electrocardiographic characteristic with abrupt V3 transition.[61]

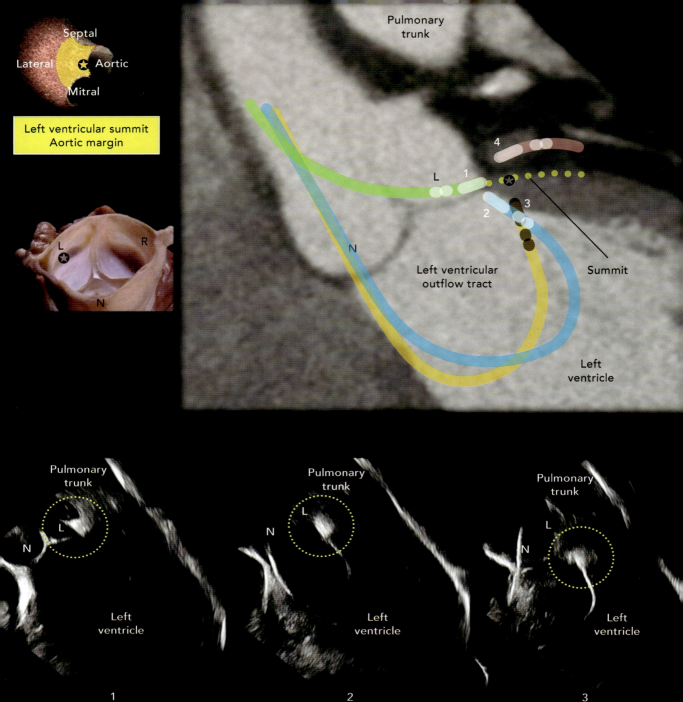

Figure 5-33 ▶ **and Figure 5-34** **Four angles of attack for left ventricular summit ventricular arrhythmia.**

There are four common vantage points: 1) retrograde approach in the left coronary aortic sinus to abla the myocardial crescent (Figure 5-27); 2) retrograde subvalvular approach with small "hockey stick" c or modified small U-turn approach to target the region just beneath the leaflet; 3) retrograde subvalvu approach with large "prolapse" curl to target endocardial aspect of the left ventricular summit; a 4) epicardial approach via the coronary venous system.

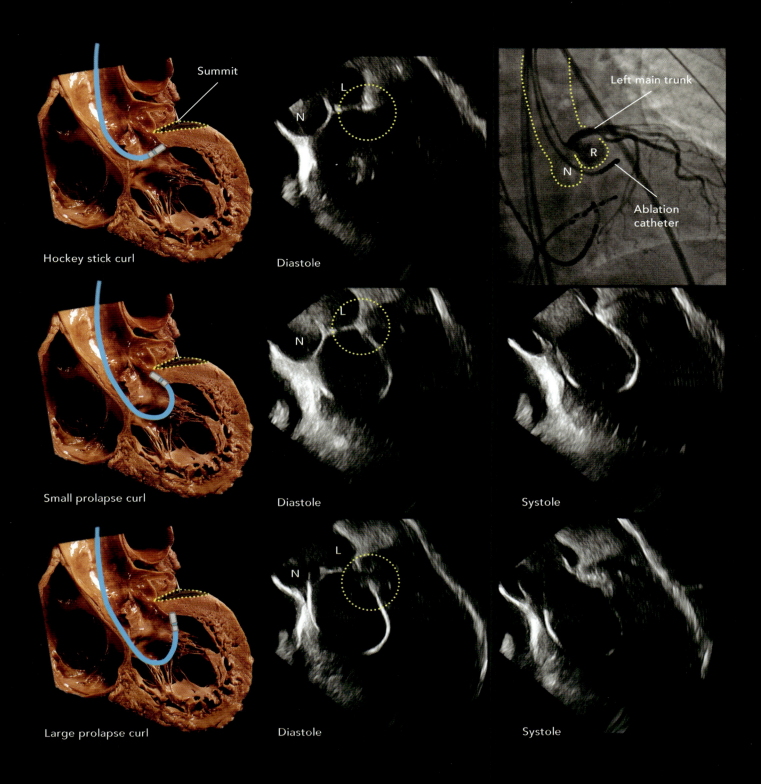

Hockey stick curl

Diastole

Left main trunk

Ablation catheter

Small prolapse curl

Diastole

Systole

Large prolapse curl

Diastole

Systole

Upper panels show a retrograde subvalvular approach with short "hockey stick" curls. Middle panels show a retrograde subvalvular approach with a small U-turn curve to target the area immediately beneath the hinge line of the left coronary aortic leaflet. The bottom panels show a larger prolapse curl to reach the corresponding endocardial aspect of the left ventricular summit.

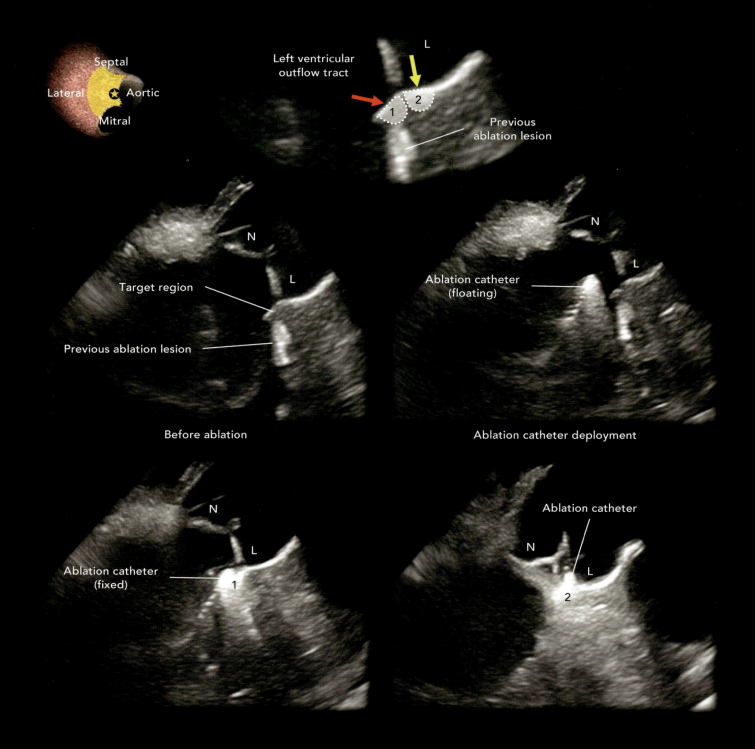

Figure 5-35 ▶ **Intracardiac echocardiography-guided ablation of a left ventricular summit arrhythmia.**

The use of intracardiac echocardiography is highlighted in this case, which had a prior failed ablation targeting the aortic margin of the left ventricular summit. Increased echogenicity indicates the previous ablation lesion, which left a gap between the leaflet hinge line. A retrogradely advanced prolapsed catheter is placed in parallel to the myocardium. Ablation from this vantage point eliminated the ventricular arrhythmia (site 1). Additional ablation was performed from the left coronary aortic sinus to reinforce the ablation effect (site 2).

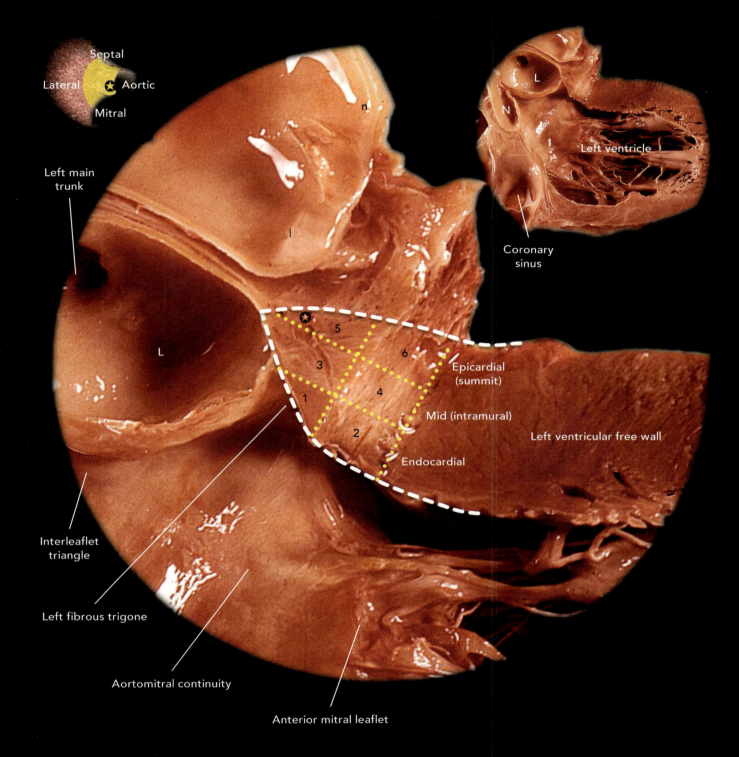

Figure 5-36 **Six-segment model of the left ventricular summit region.**

Beak-shaped sectional area involving the summit is divided into six segments. The true left ventricular summit is sites 5 and 6. Endocardial approaches that are immediately under the left coronary aortic sinus are ideal for sites 1 and 2, with the need to contact the myocardium below the leaflet. Sites 3 and 4 represent intramural sites of origin, where the left coronary aortic sinus provides the optimal vantage point into site 3. Site 4 is often the most difficult to eliminate as it is equidistant from the aforementioned vantage points (Figure 5-31).

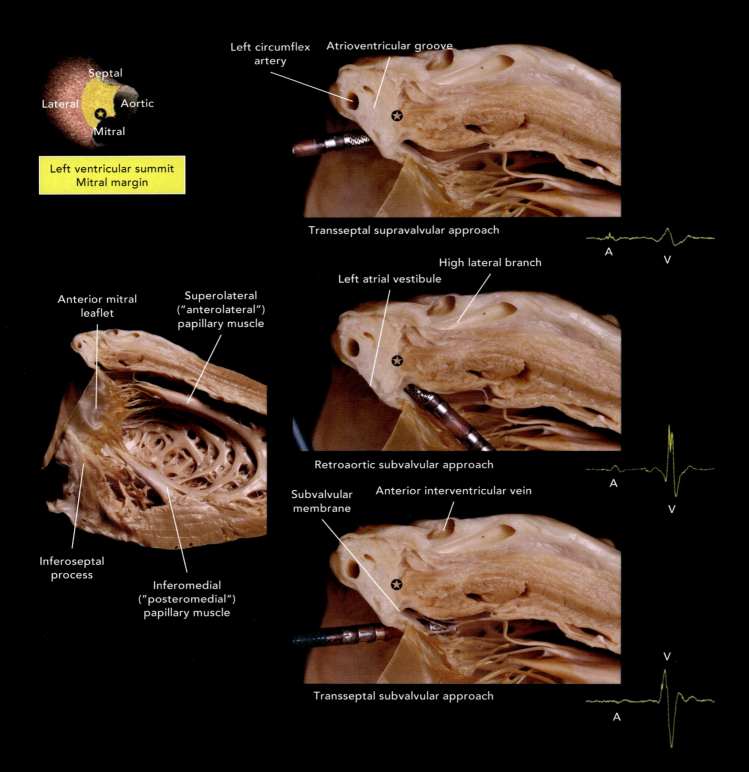

Figures 5-37 Mitral margin of the left ventricular summit.

Supravalvular far-field ventricular potential mapping (upper) is feasible to estimate the focus without inducing ventricular arrhythmias.[62] As the epicardial surface of the basal left ventricle faces the left atrial vestibule, intervened by the left atrioventricular groove, supravalvular ablation can work to ablate ventricular arrhythmia.[63] Retroaortic subvalvular (middle) and transseptal subvalvular (bottom) approaches are also demonstrated. Before supravalvular ablation, coronary angiography is necessary to confirm the left circumflex artery course.

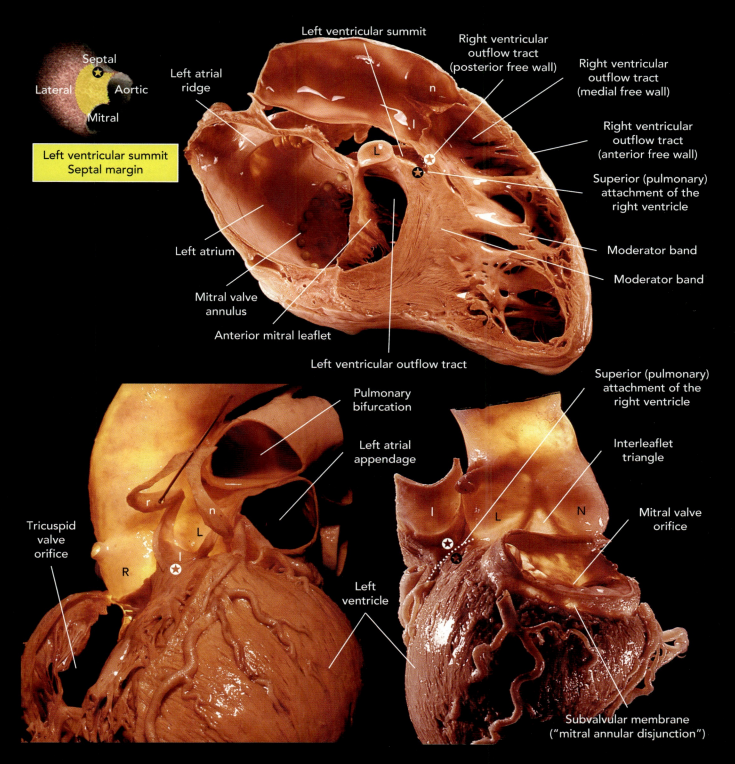

Left ventricular summit

Right ventricular outflow tract (posterior free wall)

Right ventricular outflow tract (medial free wall)

Right ventricular outflow tract (anterior free wall)

Superior (pulmonary) attachment of the right ventricle

Moderator band

Moderator band

Left atrial ridge

Left atrium

Mitral valve annulus

Anterior mitral leaflet

Left ventricular outflow tract

Septal

Lateral · Aortic

Mitral

Left ventricular summit
Septal margin

Pulmonary bifurcation

Left atrial appendage

Left ventricle

Tricuspid valve orifice

Superior (pulmonary) attachment of the right ventricle

Interleaflet triangle

Mitral valve orifice

Subvalvular membrane ("mitral annular disjunction")

Figures 5-38   Septal margin of the left ventricular summit.

The superior attachment of the right ventricle, posterior free wall of the right ventricle (white star), and left adjacent pulmonary sinus (Figure 5-24, Figure 5-28) are vantage points for the septal margin of the left ventricular summit (black star).

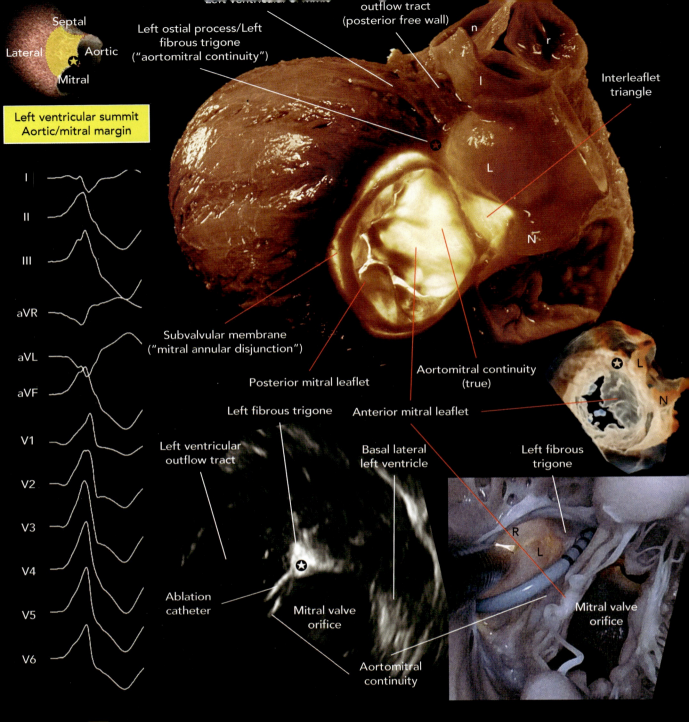

Septal
Lateral Aortic
Mitral

Left ventricular summit
Aortic/mitral margin

Left ostial process/Left fibrous trigone ("aortomitral continuity")

outflow tract (posterior free wall)

Interleaflet triangle

Subvalvular membrane ("mitral annular disjunction")

Posterior mitral leaflet

Left fibrous trigone

Left ventricular outflow tract

Ablation catheter

Aortomitral continuity (true)

Anterior mitral leaflet

Basal lateral left ventricle

Left fibrous trigone

Mitral valve orifice

Aortomitral continuity

Mitral valve orifice

I, II, III, aVR, aVL, aVF, V1, V2, V3, V4, V5, V6

Figure 5-39 ▶ **Left ostial process and left fibrous trigone.**

The angle created between the septal and mitral margins of the left ventricular summit is referred to as the left ostial process, which is also the location of the left fibrous trigone on the endocardial side. This region was referred to as the "aortomitral continuity" in the field of electrophysiology.[64] However, the aortomitral continuity is the fibrous region extending at the base of the anterior mitral leaflet without myocardial connection. An endoscopic image identical to the intracardiac echocardiography image shows a U-turn ablation of this region (bottom).

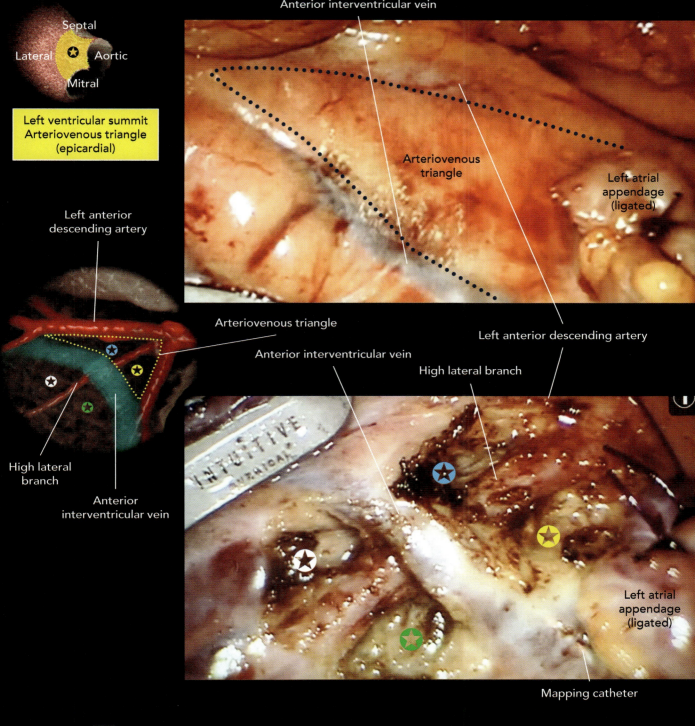

Figure 5-40 ▶ **Endoscopic robotic visualization of the left ventricular summit.**

The junction between the great cardiac vein and anterior interventricular vein, with a diagnostic catheter within, is shown. The epicardium is covered by adipose tissue and the left anterior descending artery is not directly visualized without further dissection (upper). The left atrial appendage is ligated to visualize the coronary vessels. After dissection, four quadrants demarcated by the anterior interventricular vein and high lateral branch are visualized (colored stars within the bottom panel).

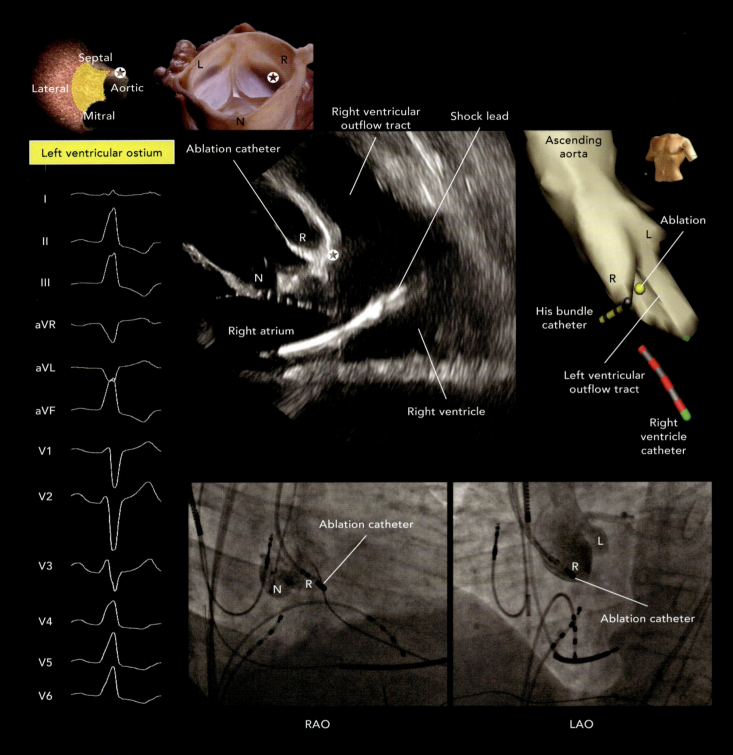

Left ventricular ostium

Septal
Lateral — Aortic
Mitral

L
R
N

I
II
III
aVR
aVL
aVF
V1
V2
V3
V4
V5
V6

Ablation catheter

Right ventricular outflow tract

Shock lead

R
N

Right atrium

Ascending aorta

Ablation

L
R

His bundle catheter

Left ventricular outflow tract

Right ventricle catheter

Right ventricle

Ablation catheter

N R

Ablation catheter

L
R

RAO

LAO

Figure 5-41 ▶ *Spotlight:* **Ablation from the right coronary aortic sinus.**

The right coronary aortic sinus is the most anterior sinus of the aortic root. It shares the basal septal myocardium with the septal right ventricular outflow tract beneath the ventriculoarterial junction. Above the junction, the posterolateral free wall of the right ventricular outflow tract covers the right coronary aortic sinus. Ventricular arrhythmias originating from the myocardial crescent typically show a left bundle branch block morphology with a transition zone around V3.

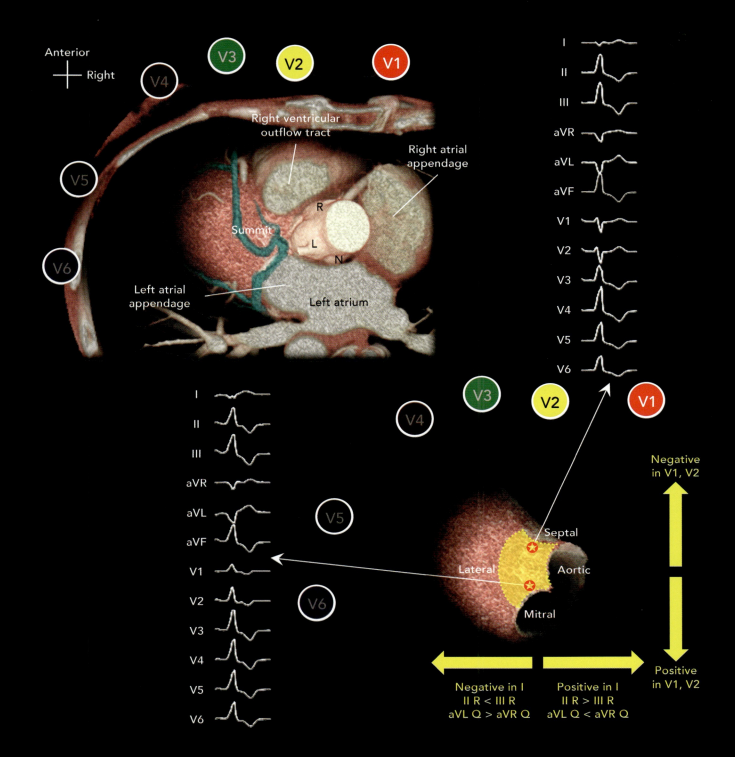

Figure 5-42 Relationship between the left ventricular summit and precordial leads.

Left ventricular summit arrhythmia shows marked QRS variations even within this confined area. Anatomical understanding is the key to estimating the focus of a given arrhythmia. As it gets closer to the V1 and V2, the septal side may yield left bundle branch block QRS morphologies with abrupt V3 transition,[61] whereas the mitral side typically shows R-wave concordance with wider QRS width. Note the identical deflections recorded in the limb leads. As the focus is lateral to the left coronary aortic sinus, generally II R < III R, and aVL Q > aVR Q.

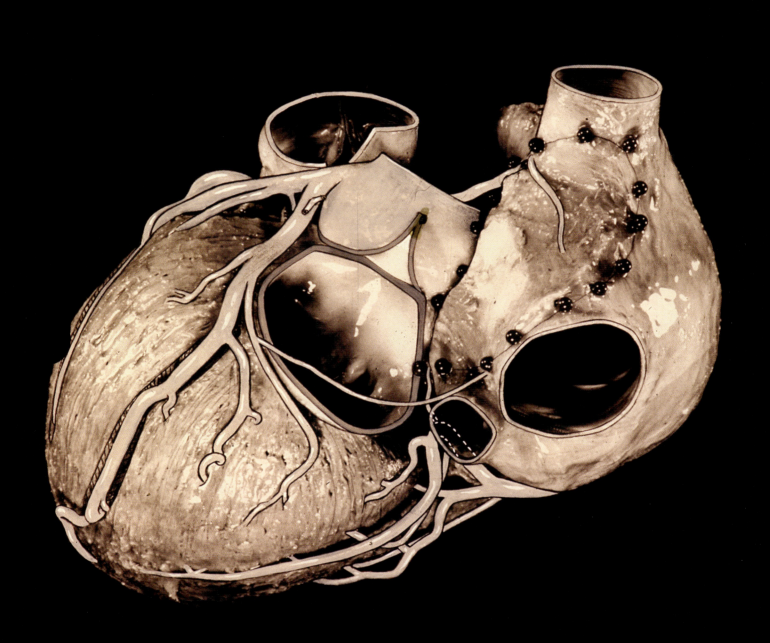

Resources and References

Resources

McAlpine WA. *Heart and Coronary Arteries: An Anatomical Atlas for Clinical Diagnosis, Radiological Investigation, and Surgical Treatment.* Springer-Verlag; 1975.

Mori S, Shivkumar K. *Atlas of Cardiac Anatomy (Anatomical Basis of Cardiac Interventions. Vol. 1).* Cardiotext; 2022.

References

1. Mori S, Hanna P, Dacey MJ, Temma T, Hadaya J, Zhu C, et al. Comprehensive anatomy of the pericardial space and the cardiac hilum: Anatomical dissections with intact. *JACC Cardiovasc Imaging.* 2022;15(5):927–942.

2. Mori S, Tretter JT, Spicer DE, Bolender DL, Anderson RH. What is the real cardiac anatomy? *Clin Anat.* 2019;32(3):288–309.

3. Mori S, Fukuzawa K, Takaya T, Takamine S, Ito T, Fujiwara S, et al. Clinical cardiac structural anatomy reconstructed within the cardiac contour using multidetector-row computed tomography: Left ventricular outflow tract. *Clin Anat.* 2016;29(3):353–363.

4. Sato T, Adlaka K, Moussa ID, Hanna P, Do DH, Fishbein MC, et al. Understanding cardiac anatomy and imaging to improve safety of procedures: The right ventricle. *JACC Cardiovasc Imaging.* 2023;16(10):1348–1352.

5. Mori S, Fukuzawa K, Takaya T, Takamine S, Ito T, Fujiwara S, et al. Clinical cardiac structural anatomy reconstructed within the cardiac contour using multidetector-row computed tomography: Atrial septum and ventricular septum. *Clin Anat.* 2016;29(3):342–352.

6. Mori S, Fukuzawa K, Takaya T, Takamine S, Ito T, Fujiwara S, et al. Clinical structural anatomy of the inferior pyramidal space reconstructed within the cardiac using multidetector-row computed tomography. *J Cardiovasc Electrophysiol.* 2015;26(7):705–712.

7. Mori S, Fukuzawa K, Takaya T, Takamine S, Ito T, Fujiwara S, et al. Clinical cardiac structural anatomy reconstructed within the cardiac contour using multidetector-row computed tomography: The arrangement and location of the cardiac valves. *Clin Anat.* 2016;29(3):364–370.

8. Mori S, Fukuzawa K, Takaya T, Takamine S, Ito T, Kinugasa M, et al. Optimal angulations for obtaining an en face view of each coronary aortic sinus and the interventricular septum: Correlative anatomy around the left ventricular outflow tract. *Clin Anat.* 2015;28(4):494–505.

9. Nakahara S, Ramirez RJ, Buch E, Michowitz Y, Vaseghi M, de Diego C, et al. Intrapericardial balloon placement for prevention of collateral injury during catheter ablation of the left atrium in a porcine model. *Heart Rhythm.* 2010;7(1):81–87.

10. Khakpour H, Mori S, Bradfield JS, Shivkumar K. How to use intracardiac echocardiography to recognize normal cardiac anatomy. *Card Electrophysiol Clin.* 2021;13(2):273–283.

11. Armour JA, Murphy DA, Yuan B-X, MacDonald S, Hopkins DA. Gross and microscopic anatomy of the human intrinsic cardiac nervous system. *The Anatomical Record.* 1997;247(2):289–298.

12. Al Aloul B, Sigurdsson G, Can I, Li JM, Dykoski R, Tholakanahalli VN. Proximity of right coronary artery to cavotricuspid isthmus as determined by computed tomography. *Pacing Clin Electrophysiol.* 2010;33(11):1319–1323.

13. Mykytsey A, Kehoe R, Bharati S, Maheshwari P, Halleran S, Krishnan K, et al. Right coronary artery occlusion during RF ablation of typical atrial flutter. *J Cardiovasc Electrophysiol.* 2010;21(7):818–821.

14. Mori S, Nishii T, Takaya T, Kashio K, Kasamatsu A, Takamine S, et al. Clinical structural anatomy of the inferior pyramidal space reconstructed from the living heart: Three-dimensional visualization using multidetector-row computed tomography. *Clin Anat*. 2015;28(7):878–888

15. Anderson RH, Sanchez-Quintana D, Mori S, Spicer DE, Wellens HJJ, Lokhwandala Y, et al. Miniseries 2-Septal and paraseptal accessory pathways-Part I: The anatomic basis for the understanding of para-Hisian accessory atrio-ventricular pathways. *Europace*. 2022;24(4):639–649.

16. Mori S, Anderson RH, Takaya T, Toba T, Ito T, Fujiwara S, et al. The association between wedging of the aorta and cardiac structural anatomy as revealed using multidetector-row computed tomography. *J Anat*. 2017;231(1):110–1120.

17. Mori S, Moussa ID, Hanna P, Shivkumar K. Veiled anatomy of the tricuspid valve perimeter: What the interventionalist must know . . . but cannot see! *JACC Cardiovasc Interv*. 2023;16(5):614–616.

18. Mori S, Hanna P, Bhatt RV, Shivkumar K. The atrioventricular bundle: A sesquicentennial tribute to Professor Sunao Tawara. *JACC Clin Electrophysiol*. 2023;9(3):444–447.

19. Tavares L, Dave A, Valderrabano M. Successful ablation of premature ventricular contractions originating from the inferoseptal process of the left ventricle using a coronary sinus approach. *Heart Rhythm Case Rep*. 2018;4(8):371–374.

20. Santangeli P, Hyman MC, Muser D, Callans DJ, Shivkumar K, Marchlinski FE. Outcomes of percutaneous trans-right atrial access to the left ventricle for catheter ablation of ventricular tachycardia in patients with mechanical aortic and mitral valves. *JAMA Cardiol*. 2020;6(3):1–6.

21. Gerbode F, Hultgren H, Melrose D, Osborn J. Syndrome of left ventricular-right atrial shunt: Successful surgical repair of defect in five cases, with observation of bradycardia on closure. *Ann Surg*. 1958;148(3):433–446.

22. Can I, Krueger K, Chandrashekar Y, Li JM, Dykoski R, Tholakanahalli VN. Images in cardiovascular medicine. Gerbode-type defect induced by catheter ablation of the atrioventricular node. *Circulation*. 2009;119(22):e553–e556.

23. Zaidi SMJ, Sohail H, Satti DI, Sami A, Anwar M, Malik J, et al. Tricuspid regurgitation in His bundle pacing: A systematic review. *Ann Noninvasive Electrocardiol*. 2022;27(6):e12986.

24. Rizkallah J, Burgess J, Kuriachan V. Absent right and persistent left superior vena cava: Troubleshooting during a challenging pacemaker implant: A case report. *BMC Res Notes*. 2014;7:462.

25. Wissner E, Tilz R, Konstantinidou M, Metzner A, Schmidt B, Chun KR, et al. Catheter ablation of atrial fibrillation in patients with persistent left superior vena cava is associated with major intraprocedural complications. *Heart Rhythm*. 2010;7(12):1755–1760.

26. Sadek MM, Benhayon D, Sureddi R, Chik W, Santangeli P, Supple GE, et al. Idiopathic ventricular arrhythmias originating from the moderator band: Electrocardiographic characteristics and treatment by catheter ablation. *Heart Rhythm*. 2015;12(1):67–75.

27. Dong X, Tang M, Sun Q, Zhang S. Anatomical relevance of ablation to the pulmonary artery root: Clinical implications for characterizing the pulmonary sinus of Valsalva and coronary artery. *J Cardiovasc Electrophysiol*. 2018;29(9):1230–1237.

28. Liao Z, Zhan X, Wu S, Xue Y, Fang X, Liao H, et al. Idiopathic ventricular arrhythmias originating from the pulmonary sinus cusp: Prevalence, electrocardiographic/electrophysiological characteristics, and catheter ablation. *J Am Coll Cardiol*. 2015;66(23):2633–2644.

29. Anderson RH, Mori S, Spicer DE, Cheung JW, Lerman BB. Living anatomy of the pulmonary root. *J Cardiovasc Electrophysiol*. 2018;29(9):1238–1240.

30. Futyma P, Moroka K, Derndorfer M, Kollias G, Martinek M, Purerfellner H. Left pulmonary cusp ablation of refractory ventricular arrhythmia originating from the inaccessible summit. *Europace*. 2019;21(8):1253.

31. Hayase J, Shapiro H, Bae D, Shantouf R, Wachsner R. Dual chamber pacemaker implantation complicated by left anterior descending coronary artery injury. *JACC Case Rep*. 2019;1(4):633–637.

32. Yokokawa M, Good E, Chugh A, Pelosi F, Jr., Crawford T, Jongnarangsin K, et al. Intramural idiopathic ventricular arrhythmias originating in the intraventricular septum: Mapping and ablation. *Circ Arrhythm Electrophysiol*. 2012;5(2):258–263.

33. Romero J, Diaz JC, Hayase J, Dave RH, Bradfield JS, Shivkumar K. Intramyocardial radiofrequency ablation of ventricular arrhythmias using intracoronary wire mapping and a coronary reentry system: Description of a novel technique. *Heart Rhythm Case Rep.* 2018;4(7):285–292.

34. Patel A, Nsahlai M, Flautt T, Da-Warikobo A, Lador A, Tapias C, et al. Advanced techniques for ethanol ablation of left ventricular summit region arrhythmias. *Circ Arrhythm Electrophysiol.* 2022;15(8):e011017.

35. Trivedi R, Rattigan E, Bauch TD, Mascarenhas V, Ahmad T, Subzposh FA, Vijayaraman P. Giant interventricular septal hematoma complicating left bundle branch pacing: A cautionary tale. *JACC Case Rep.* 2023;16:101887.

36. Mori S, Bradfield JS. Ventricular arrhythmias ablated from the noncoronary aortic sinus: Underrecognized myocardium of the right ventricle. *JACC Clin Electrophysiol.* 2023;9(8 Pt 1):1292–1295.

37. Tretter JT, Mori S, Saremi F, Chikkabyrappa S, Thomas K, Bu F, et al. Variations in rotation of the aortic root and membranous septum with implications for transcatheter valve implantation. *Heart.* 2018;104(12):999–1005.

38. Liao Z, Dai S, Nie Z, Song X, Huang X, Wang J, et al. Reappraisal and new observations on idiopathic ventricular arrhythmias ablated from the noncoronary aortic sinus. *JACC Clin Electrophysiol.* 2023;9(8 Pt 1):1279–1291.

39. Yamamoto K, Mori S, Fukuzawa K, Miyamoto K, Toba T, Izawa Y, et al. Revisiting the prevalence and diversity of localized thinning of the left ventricular apex. *J Cardiovasc Electrophysiol.* 2020;31(4):915–920.

40. Merrick AF, Yacoub MH, Ho SY, Anderson RH. Anatomy of the muscular subpulmonary infundibulum with regard to the Ross procedure. *Ann Thorac Surg.* 2000;69(2):556–561.

41. Marshall J. On the development of the great anterior veins in man and mammalia; including an account of certain remnants of foetal structure found in the adult, a comparative view of these great veins in the different mammalia, and an analysis of their occasional peculiarities in the human subject. *Phil Trans Royal Soc London.* 1850;140:133–170.

42. Kim DT, Lai AC, Hwang C, Fan LT, Karagueuzian HS, Chen PS, Fishbein MC. The ligament of Marshall: A structural analysis in human hearts with implications for atrial arrhythmias. *J Am Coll Cardiol.* 2000;36(4):1324–1327.

43. Hwang C, Chen PS. Ligament of Marshall: Why it is important for atrial fibrillation ablation. *Heart Rhythm.* 2009;6(12 Suppl):S35–S40.

44. Esrailian DL, Mori S, Shivkumar K. Understanding cardiac anatomy and imaging to improve safety of procedures: The sinus node artery. *JACC Case Rep.* 2023;28:102124.

45. Jiang R, Buch E, Gima J, Upadhyay GA, Nayak HM, Beaser AD, et al. Feasibility of percutaneous epicardial mapping and ablation for refractory atrial fibrillation: Insights into substrate and lesion transmurality. *Heart Rhythm.* 2019;16(8):1151–1159.

46. Rao S, Kwasnik A, Tung R. Direct epicardial recordings in the region of the septopulmonary bundle: Anatomy "behind" posterior wall activation. *JACC Clin Electrophysiol.* 2020;6(9):1214–1216.

47. Vaseghi M, Macias C, Tung R, Shivkumar K. Percutaneous interventricular septal access in a patient with aortic and mitral mechanical valves: A novel technique for catheter ablation of ventricular tachycardia. *Heart Rhythm.* 2013;10(7):1069–1073.

48. Sato T, Moussa ID, Hanna P, Shivkumar K, Mori S. Intermediate accessory papillary muscle: An anatomic variant of interest for transcatheter edge-to-edge mitral valve repair. *Circ Cardiovasc Imaging.* 2023;16(10):e015151.

49. Tawara S. Das Reizleitungssystem Des Säugetierherzens. Eine Anatomisch-Histologische Studie Über das Atrioventrikularbündel und die Purkinjeschen Fäden. Jena: Gustav Fischer. 1906.

50. Vijayaraman P, Chelu MG, Curila K, Dandamudi G, Herweg B, Mori S, et al. Cardiac conduction system pacing: A comprehensive update. *JACC Clin Electrophysiol.* 2023;9(11):2358–2387.

51. Liang JJ, Shirai Y, Briceno DF, Muser D, Enriquez A, Lin A, et al. Electrocardiographic and electrophysiologic characteristics of idiopathic ventricular arrhythmias originating from the basal inferoseptal left ventricle. *JACC Clin Electrophysiol.* 2019;5(7):833–842.

52. Kawamura M, Gerstenfeld EP, Vedantham V, Rodrigues DM, Burkhardt JD, Kobayashi Y, et al. Idiopathic ventricular arrhythmia originating from the cardiac crux or inferior septum: Epicardial idiopathic ventricular arrhythmia. *Circ Arrhythm Electrophysiol.* 2014;7(6):1152–1158.

53. Wilber DJ, Kopp DE, Glascock DN, Kinder CA, Kall JG. Catheter ablation of the mitral isthmus for ventricular tachycardia associated with inferior infarction. *Circulation.* 1995;92(12):3481–3489.

54. Martinov E, Marchov D, Marinov M, Boychev D, Gelev V, Traykov V. Endocardial, epicardial, and right atrial approach for catheter ablation of premature ventricular contractions from the inferoseptal process of the left ventricle. *J Arrhythm.* 2023;39(4):613–620.

55. Yamada T, Doppalapudi H, McElderry HT, Okada T, Murakami Y, Inden Y, et al. Electrocardiographic and electrophysiological characteristics in idiopathic ventricular arrhythmias originating from the papillary muscles in the left ventricle: Relevance for catheter ablation. *Circ Arrhythm Electrophysiol.* 2010;3(4):324–331.

56. Enriquez A, Supple GE, Marchlinski FE, Garciaf FC. How to map and ablate papillary muscle ventricular arrhythmias. *Heart Rhythm.* 2017;14(11):1721–1728.

57. Komatsu Y, Nogami A, Kurosaki K, Morishima I, Masuda K, Ozawa T, et al. Fascicular ventricular tachycardia originating from papillary muscles: Purkinje network involvement in the reentrant circuit. *Circ Arrhythm Electrophysiol.* 2017;10(3).

58. Mori S, Bradfield JS, Fukuzawa K, Shivkumar K. Comprehensive anatomy of the summit of the left ventricle. *JACC Clin Electrophysiol.* 2024;10(1):168–184.

59. Yamada T, McElderry HT, Doppalapudi H, Okada T, Murakami Y, Yoshida Y, et al. Idiopathic ventricular arrhythmias originating from the left ventricular summit: Anatomic concepts relevant to ablation. *Circ Arrhythm Electrophysiol.* 2010;3(6):616–623.

60. Sato T, Bradifield JS, Shivkumar K, Mori S. Understanding cardiac anatomy and imaging to improve safety of procedures: The interleaflet triangle. *JACC Clin Electrophysiol.* Published online February 2, 2024. doi:10.1016/j.jacep.2024.01.010

61. Liao H, Wei W, Tanager KS, Miele F, Upadhyay GA, Beaser AD, et al. Left ventricular summit arrhythmias with an abrupt V(3) transition: Anatomy of the aortic interleaflet triangle vantage point. *Heart Rhythm.* 2021;18(1):10–19.

62. Nakasone K, Mori S, Izawa Y, Kiuchi K, Takami M, Hirata KI, Fukuzawa K. Transseptal Supravalvular supravalvular far-field potential mapping of ventricular premature contractions originating around the superior mitral annulus. *JACC Clin Electrophysiol.* 2023;9(9):2034–2039.

63. Yamagami S, Mori S, Nishiuchi S, Akiyama M, Nakano Y, Kondo H, et al. Successful supravalvular radiofrequency catheter ablation of premature ventricular contractions originating from the left ventricular summit. *JACC Clin Electrophysiol.* 2024;10(2):405–413.

64. Steven D, Roberts-Thomson KC, Seiler J, Inada K, Tedrow UB, Mitchell RN, et al. Ventricular tachycardia arising from the aortomitral continuity in structural heart disease: Characteristics and therapeutic considerations for an anatomically challenging area of origin. *Circ Arrhythm Electrophysiol.* 2009;2(6):660–666.